Clinica
Cancer

C000134046

A Companion to *Cancer Nursing,* Fifth Edition

Edited by
....

Connie Henke Yarbro, RN, MS, FAAN
Editor, *Seminars in Oncology Nursing*
Clinical Associate Professor, Division of Hematology/Oncology, Adjunct Clinical Assistant Professor, MU Sinclair School of Nursing, University of Missouri, Columbia, Columbia, Missouri

Margaret Hansen Frogge, RN, MS
Vice President—Strategic Development, Rush-Riverside Cancer Center, Riverside Medical Center, Kankakee, IL. Assistant Professor, Rush University College of Nursing, Chicago, Illinois

Michelle Goodman, RN, MS
Assistant Professor of Nursing, Rush University College of Nursing, Oncology Clinical Nurse Specialist, Section of Medical Oncology, Rush Cancer Institute, Rush-Presbyterian-St. Luke's Medical Center, Chicago, Illinois

JONES AND BARTLETT PUBLISHERS
Sudbury, Massachusetts
BOSTON   TORONTO   LONDON   SINGAPORE

World Headquarters

Jones and Bartlett
Publishers
40 Tall Pine Drive
Sudbury, MA 01776
(978) 443-5000
Info@jbpub.com
http://www.jbpub.com

Jones and Bartlett
Publishers Canada
2406 Nikanna Road
Mississauga, ON L5C 2W6
Canada

Jones and Bartlett
Publishers International
Barb House, Barb Mews
London W6 7PA
UK

Acquisitions Editor: Penny Glynn
Associate Editor: Thomas Prindle
Production Editor: Jon Workman
Marketing Manager: Taryn Wahlquist
Manufacturing Buyer: Amy Duddridge
Editorial and Production Service: Colophon
Composition: Modern Graphics
Printing and Binding: Courier Westford
Cover Design: Philip Regan

Library of Congress Cataloging-in-Publication Data
CIP data is unavailable at time of printing.

The selection and dosage of drugs presented in this
book are in accord with standards accepted at the
time of publication. The editors and the publisher
have made every effort to provide accurate
information. However, research, clinical practice, and
government regulations often change the accepted
standard in this field. Before administering any drug,
the reader is advised to check the manufacturer's
product information sheet for the most up-to-date
recommendations on dosage, precautions, and
contraindications. This is especially important in the
case of drugs that are new or seldom used.

Printed in the United States of America.
05 04 03 02 01   10 9 8 7 6 5 4 3 2 1

Contents

The Editors

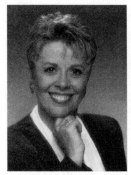

Connie Henke Yarbro

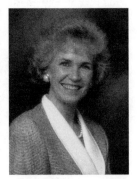

Margaret Hansen Frogge

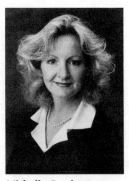

Michelle Goodman

Preface

In our continuing commitment to provide resources to all nurses who care for individuals with cancer, we designed *Clinical Guide to Cancer Nursing* as an easy-to-use nursing reference. Information most pertinent to the care of individuals with cancer has been gleaned from *Cancer Nursing: Principles and Practice, Fifth Edition,* and consolidated in this pocket-size clinical reference.

The content of this clinical guide includes selected chapters from *Cancer Nursing: Principles and Practice, 5th edition.* Content has been thoroughly updated throughout and is presented in an abbreviated format to enhance the readability and aid in locating desired information quickly.

Part I, The Cancer Problem, covers epidemiology and pathophysiology of cancer. Content on the biology of cancer has been completely updated to reflect the latest research. Part II, Prevention, Detection, and Diagnosis discusses the dynamics of cancer prevention, chemoprevention, diagnostics, and a chapter on genetic risk and counseling. Part III, Treatment, outlines standard and emerging treatment modalities, including a new chapter on gene therapy. Part IV, Symptom Management, provides step-by-step management of common symptoms in cancer patients. Chapters are alphabetized by subject. Part V, Oncologic Emergencies, is a new section that focuses on the management and care of these acute symptoms. Part VI, The Care of Individuals with Cancer, details the specific medical and nursing management for patients with 27 specific types of cancer. And finally, we have provided two appendixes on Oral Antineoplastic Agents and Intravenous Antineoplastic Agents.

For more comprehensive information on the subject and references, the reader is referred to chapters in *Cancer Nursing: Principles and Practice* 5th Edition from which the content was extrapolated.

We sincerely hope that this book will be an easy-to-use, quick, and helpful reference to nurses—wherever they are caring for patients with cancer.

Acknowledgments

Our special thanks to the nurses who continue to provide us with feedback, suggestions, and encouragement regarding the information and resources they need in caring for patients with cancer. Thanks to Jones and Bartlett Publishers for their assistance and their commitment to providing quality textbooks to oncology nurses. Finally, we acknowledge and thank the following authors whose chapters in *Cancer Nursing: Principles and Practice, Fifth Edition* were used to derive the content contained in this guide:

Terri Ades, RN, CS, MS, AOCN
Director, Health Content
American Cancer Society, Inc.
Atlanta, GA

Linda Battiato, RN, MSN, OCN®
Oncology/Cytokine Research Nurse
Indiana Cancer Pavilion
Indianapolis, IN

Susan M. Bauer, DNSc, RN
Assistant Professor
Graduate School of Nursing and
    Division of Preventive & Behavioral
    Medicine
University of Massachusetts
    Worcester/University of
    Massachusetts Medical Center
Worcester, MA

Susan Weiss Behrend, RN, MSN
Oncology Clinical Nurse Specialist
Fox Chase Cancer Center
Philadelphia, PA

Karen Belford, RN, MS, AOCN, CCRN
Nurse Educator
Memorial Sloan-Kettering Cancer
    Center
Department of Nursing Education
New York, NY

Dawn Camp-Sorrell, RN, MSN, FNP, AOCN
Oncology Nurse Practitioner
Central Alabama Hematology
    Oncology Associates
Birmingham, AL

Dianne D. Chapman, RN, MS
Coordinator
Comprehensive Breast Center
Chicago, IL

JoAnn Coleman, RN, MS, ACNP-CS, AOCN
Acute Care Nurse Practitioner
Pancreas and Biliary Surgery
Johns Hopkins Hospital
Baltimore, MD

Shawanna M. Cunning, RN, MSN, CCRN
Clinical Nurse Specialist
Riverside Medical Center
Kankakee, IL

Lynne M. Early, RN, MSN, CETN, OCN®
Enterostomal Therapy Nurse
Los Angeles, CA

Jan Ellerhorst-Ryan, RN, MSN, CS
Oncology-HIV Clinical Nurse Specialist
United Home Health
Cincinnati, OH

Coni Ellis, MS, RN-CS, C, OCN®, CWOCN
Nursing Outreach Coordinator; Co-Director of the Wound, Ostomy, and Continence Nurse Education Program
The University of Texas M.D. Anderson Cancer Center
Houston, TX

Anne Marie Flaherty, RN, MSN, AOCN, CNSC
Clinical Nurse Specialist
Hackensack University Medical Center, Adult Oncology
Hackensack, NJ

Ann T. Foltz, RN, DNS
Consultant, ATF Quality Control
Leesburg, FL

Margaret Hansen Frogge, RN, MS
Vice President, Strategic Development and System Integration
Riverside Health Care
Kankakee, IL
Assistant Professor of Nursing
Rush University College of Nursing
Rush-Presbyterian-St.Luke's Medical Center
Chicago, IL

Barbara Holmes Gobel, RN, MS
Oncology Clinical Nurse Specialist
Gottlieb Memorial Hospital
Melrose Park, IL
Complementary Faculty
Rush University College of Nursing
Chicago, IL

Michelle Goodman, RN, MS
Assistant Professor of Nursing
Rush University College of Nursing
Oncology Clinical Nurse Specialist
Section of Medical Oncology
Rush Cancer Institute
Rush-Presbyterian-St. Luke's Medical Center
Chicago, IL

Jean Gribbon, RN, BSN
Staff Nurse, Pediatrics
The University of Arizona Health Sciences Center
Tucson, AZ

Jill Griffin-Brown, RN, BSN, OCN®
Nurse Manager
Bay Area Oncology
Tampa, FL

Carol Guarnieri, RN, MSN, AOCN
Oncology Clinical Nurse Specialist
Samitivej Srinakarin Hospital
Bangkok, Thailand

Irene Stewart Haapoja, RN, MS
Oncology Clinical Nurse Specialist
Section of Medical Oncology
Rush Cancer Institute
Rush-Presbyterian-St. Luke's Medical Center
Chicago, IL

Lenore L. Harris, RN, MSN, AOCN
Study Development Coordinator
American College of Surgeons
Oncology Group
Chicago, IL

Jeanne Held-Warmkessel, RN, MSN, CS, AOCN
Clinical Nurse Specialist
Fox Chase Cancer Center
Philadelphia, PA

Wendy Hobbie, RN, MSN, CRNP
Coordinator, Follow-up Program
Children's Hospital of Philadelphia
Associate Program Director
Pediatric Oncology Nurse Practitioner
    Program
Philadelphia, PA

Laura J. Hilderley, RN, MS
Clinical Nurse Specialist, Radiation
    Oncology
Radiation Oncology Services of Rhode
    Island
Warwick, RI

Rebecca J. Ingle, RN, MSN, CS, FNP
Family Nurse Practitioner
Saint Thomas Hospital
Adjunct Instructor of Nursing
Vanderbilt University School of
    Nursing
Nashville, TN

Roberta Kaplow, RN, PhD, CCNS, CCRN
Nurse Educator, Critical Care
Memorial Sloan-Kettering Cancer
    Center
Department of Nursing Education
New York, NY

Paula R. Klemm, RN, DNSc, OCN®
Associate Professor
University of Delaware, Department
    of Nursing
Newark, DE

Dale Halsey Lea, RN, MPH
Assistant Director, Southern Maine
    Genetics Services
Foundation for Blood Research
Scarborough, ME

Lois J. Loescher, PhD, RN
Senior Research Specialist
Cancer Prevention and Control
Arizona Cancer Center
Tuscon, AZ

Jean Lydon, RN, MS, AOCN
Manager Oncology Services
Christ Hospital
Oak Lawn, IL

Karen Maher, RN, MS, ANP, AOCN
Adult Nurse Practitioner
Radiation Oncology
Legacy Health System
Portland, OR

Suzanne M. Mahon, RN, DNSc, AOCN
Assistant Clinical Professor
St. Louis University, Division of
    Hematology and Oncology
St. Louis, MO

Virginia R. Martin, MSN, RN, AOCN
Clinical Director, Ambulatory Care
Fox Chase Cancer Center
Philadelphia, PA

Mary Maxwell, RN, PhD
Clinical Specialist/Nurse Practitioner
    in Oncology
Nepal

Roxanne McDaniel, PhD, RN
Associate Professor
MU Sinclair School of Nursing
University of Missouri-Columbia
Columbia, MO

Deborah B. McGuire, PhD, RN, FAAN
Associate Professor
Director, Oncology Advanced Practice
  Nursing Program
University of Pennsylvania, School of
  Nursing
Philadelphia, PA

Ida M. (Ki) Moore, RN, DNS, FAAN
Professor and Director
Division of Nursing Practice
College of Nursing
University of Arizona
Tucson, AZ

Susan A. O'Connell, MSN, RN, OCN®
Oncology Clinical Nurse Specialist
Amgen, Inc.
Plymouth, MI

Katherine G. O'Connor, RN, MS, ANP
Nurse Practitioner, Medical Oncology
  Units
Memorial Sloan-Kettering Cancer
  Center
New York, NY

James C. Pace, DSN, RN, MDiv, ANP-CS,
Associate Professor of Adult and Elder
  Health Nursing
Nell Hodgson Woodruff School of
  Nursing
Emory University
Atlanta, GA

Jennifer Petersen RN, MS, OCN®
Oncology Clinical Nurse Specialist
Section of Medical Oncology
Rush Cancer Institute
Rush Presbyterian-St. Luke's Medical
  Center
Chicago, IL

Patricia Piasecki, RN, MS
Clinical Coordinator Orthopedic
  Oncology
Chicago, IL

Shelley M. Poirier, MS, RN, OCN®
Clinical Nurse Specialist GI Cancer
  Program
Indiana University Cancer Center
Indiana University School of Medicine
Indianapolis, IN

Rosemary Polomano, PhD, RN, FAAN
Senior Nursing Research Specialist
Center for Patient Services,
  Evaluation, Research and
  Informatics
Milton S. Hershey Medical Center
Hershey, PA

Rita M. Poquette, RN, MSN, FNP, CS
Urology Nurse Practitioner
USC/Kenneth Norris Jr. Cancer
  Hospital
Los Angeles, CA

Kathy Price, RN, OCN®
Clinical Research Specialist
Vanderbilt Cancer Center
Vanderbilt University
Nashville, TN

Susan M. Rawl, PhD, RN
Postdoctoral Fellow
Indiana University School of Nursing
Indianapolis, IN

Anita M. Reedy, RN, MSN, OCN®
Research Nurse
Johns Hopkins Oncology Center
Baltimore, MD

Mary E. Reid, PhD
Research Instructor
Co-Director, Cancer Prevention and
    Control Training Program
Arizona Cancer Center
Arizona College of Public Health
Tucson, AZ

Verna A. Rhodes, EdS, RN, FAAN
Associate Professor Emeritus
MU Sinclair School of Nursing
University of Missouri-Columbia
Columbia, MO

**Paula Trahan Rieger, RN, MSN, CS,
AOCN, FAAN**
Nurse Practitioner
Human Clinical Cancer Genetics
Department of Clinical Cancer
    Prevention
The University of Texas M.D. Anderson
    Cancer Center
Houston, TX

Mary Roach, MS, RN, AOCN
Hospice Nurse
Presbyterian Healthcare Services
Albuquerque, NM

Kimberly Rohan, MS, RN
Edward Cancer Center
Naperville, IL

**Jennifer Rychcik, MS, FNP, ACNP, CS,
CETN, OCN®**
Acute Care Nurse Practitioner
Department of Surgical Nursing
The Johns Hopkins Hospital
Baltimore, MD

**Delores Ann Hubbard Saddler, RN,
MSN, CGRN**
Clinical Care Coordinator—GI Center
University of Texas

M.D. Anderson Cancer Center
Houston, TX

Vivian R. Scheidler, MS, RN
Senior Clinical Research Scientist
Glaxo Wellcome
Research Triangle Park, NC

**Maria Serrano, RN, MSN, CS, NPC,
AOCN**
Radiation Oncology Nurse
    Practitioner
Montefiore Medical Center
Bronx, NY

**Carol A. Sheridan, RN, MSN,
AOCN**
Advanced Practice Nurse
Goldens Bridge, NY

Ellen Sitton RN, MSN, OCN®
Advanced Practice Nurse, Radiation
    Oncology & Education
USC/Kenneth Norris Jr. Cancer
    Hospital
Los Angeles, CA

Peter V. Tortorice, PharmD, BCOP
Oncology Clinical Pharmacist
Illinois Masonic Cancer Center
Maywood, IL
Oncology Pharmacy Clinical
    Coordinator
Loyola University Medical Center
Cardinal Bernardin Cancer Center
Maywood, IL

**Janet Ruth Walczak, RN, MSN,
CRNP**
Nurse Practitioner
Breast Cancer Program
Johns Hopkins Oncology Center
Baltimore, MD

Marie Bakitas Whedon, MS, ARNP, FAAN
Research Assistant Professor
Dartmouth Medical School
Palliative Care Nurse Practitioner
Norris Cotton Cancer Center
Lebanon, NH

Rita Wickham, RN, PhD, AOCN
Associate Professor
Rush College of Nursing
Oncology Clinical Nurse Specialist
Rush-Presbyterian-St. Luke's Medical
    Center
Chicago, IL

Claire R. Works, RN, MN, ARNP
Nurse Practitioner
Fred Hutchinson Cancer Research
    Center
Seattle, WA

Debra Wujcik, RN, MSN, AOCN
Director, Clinical Trials Training
and Outreach

Vanderbilt Ingram Cancer Center
Adjunct Instructor
Vanderbilt University School of
    Nursing
Nashville, TN

Susan G. Yackzan, RN, MSN, AOCN
Oncology Clinical Nurse Specialist
Lexington, KY

Connie Henke Yarbro, RN, MS, FAAN
Clinical Associate Professor
Division of Hematology/Oncology
Adjunct Clinical Associate Professor
MU Sinclair School of Nursing
Editor, *Seminars in Oncology Nursing*
University of Missouri-Columbia
Columbia, MO

Katherine A. Yeager, MS, RN
Research Project Coordinator
Rollins School of Public Health
Emory University
Atlanta, GA

Jones and Bartlett Series in Oncology

Part I

The Cancer Problem

Chapter 1
....

Biology of Cancer

Cancer results from an interaction of factors at the cellular, genetic, immunological, and environmental levels. The goals of cancer research are to

- determine the mechanisms of cancer cell development,
- determine how cancers grow and spread,
- discover the means to correct abnormal mechanisms, and
- eradicate or control cancer cell populations.

Models of Tumor Development

Theory of Clonal Evolution
Although normal cells have the same genetic makeup, carcinogens mutate one or more cells and, thus, initiate tumor progression and genetic instability. The resultant tumor represents the progeny of a single cell.

Genetic Model for Tumorigenesis
Tumor formation reflects the total accumulation of mutations rather than their specific sequence.

Transformed Cell Models
Transformed cell lines are not cancer cells but have characteristics of and are similar to malignant cells and, therefore, permit investigation of cellular processes and behavior.

There are three general mechanisms whereby normal cells can be transformed to tumor cells:

1. Spontaneous transformation to characteristics typical of cancer cells
2. Chemical/physical carcinogens and biological agents such as viruses
3. Genetic manipulation

Properties of Transformed Cells

General properties of transformed cells are cytologic changes, altered cell growth, and changes in the cell membrane.

Genetic Influences Associated with Cancer

Mutations

A mutation is a permanent change in a DNA nucleotide sequence that alters the structure of a gene and may alter its protein product.

Mutations in somatic cells become problematic when they cause increases in cell proliferation, occur early in embryogenesis, or reduce genetic stability.

Mutations may be inherited, may arise spontaneously during DNA replication, or may arise from mutagens such as environmental agents. Mutations commonly associated with cancer include point mutations and insertion and deletion mutations.

Oncogenes

Oncogenes encode proteins whose action promotes cell proliferation. A mechanism for the overexpression of oncogenes is amplification, in which the number of copies of a gene increases, resulting in overexpression of the gene product.

Classes of oncogenes are distinguished by their function. The following are examples of these broad classes:

1. Growth factors influence cell growth, differentiation, and survival by binding to specific receptors in the cell membrane. The overproduction of several growth factors is implicated in cancer development.

2. Altered growth factor receptors release proliferative signals even though no growth factor is present.

3. Oncogenes encode growth factors, growth factor receptors, nonreceptor tyrosine kinases, G-proteins, serine/threonine protein kinases, and transcription factors.

Tumor-Suppressor Genes

Tumor-suppressor genes normally suppress or negatively regulate cell proliferation by encoding proteins that block the action of growth-promoting proteins.

Mutator Genes

Mutator genes control or regulate genetic instability to ensure integrity of genetic information.

Cytogenetic Abnormalities

Cancer cells typically have an abnormal chromosome number (aneuploidy), with abnormalities in chromosomes that affect oncogenes causing overexpression.

The Cell Cycle

The cell cycle has five phases:

1. G_1 phase: The cell enlarges and synthesizes proteins.
2. S phase: The cell replicates its DNA and duplicates its chromosomes.
3. G_2 phase: The cell prepares for mitosis.
4. M phase: The cell undergoes mitosis.
5. G_0 phase: The resting phase of the cell.

The Cell Cycle and Cancer

Cancer cells have weak or deficient cell cycle checkpoints, leading to instability of the human genome, survival of genetically damaged cells, and clonal evolution.

Apoptosis

Apoptosis is referred to as programmed cell death and is essential for the normal development of multicellular organisms. Apoptotic cells activate endogenous proteases, which digest the cell from the inside out and control degradation of the cell. Impaired apoptosis may be a significant factor in the etiology of cancer.

Metastasis

Metastasis is the major cause of cancer death. It is the spread of tumor cells from the primary site, via the blood stream or lymphatic system, to a distant site. The factors contributing to metastasis include:

- Angiogenesis is the formation of a new blood supply and involves the migration and proliferation of endothelial cells.
- The degree of angiogenesis in the primary tumor site correlates with metastatic potential and may be a prognostic factor.
- Motility factors are produced by tumor cells and are a primary factor in the process of metastasis.
- Cancer cells have an increased ability to break off from the primary tumor due to a lack of cell surface adhesion molecules.
- Tumor cells secrete a number of proteinases that assist with degradation of barriers to metastasis. The ratio of proteolytic enzymes to their inhibitors determines tumor invasiveness.
- Tumor cells hide from the immune system by releasing soluble antigens or intracellular adhesion molecules that block cell interactions.
- The metastatic cascade includes
  1. detachment,
  2. invasion,
  3. survival in transport,
  4. arrest in distant organ capillary bed, and
  5. establishment of secondary tumor.

Chapter 2
....

Immunology

Cancer diagnosis and treatment are related directly to immune function. An inadequate immune system may be associated with cancer development. Certain cancer therapies induce immunosuppression, while other therapies enhance the body's own immune system to fight cancer. The immune system recognizes foreign substances (antigens) and eliminates the substances through initiation of the immune response. There are two types of immune responses:

1. *Innate immunity* provides an inflammatory response and phagocytosis of the foreign substance.
2. *Adaptive* or *acquired immunity* forms the basis of vaccination to control certain diseases.

Components of the Immune System

Structures of the Immune System
The primary lymphoid organs include the bone marrow, which produces B cells, and the thymus, which produces T cells. Secondary lymphoid organs include the spleen, lymph nodes, tonsils, Peyer's patches in the gastrointestinal tract, and the bone marrow.

Cells of the Immune System
Leukocytes arise from the bone marrow and give rise to myeloid and lymphoid cell lines.

- The *myeloid lineage* produces monocytes, polymorphonuclear leukocytes, and platelets. These cells function as phagocytic macrophages, removing particulate antigens.

- The *lymphoid lineage* produces B lymphocytes, T lymphocytes, and natural killer cells. B cells are antibody-secreting plasma cells. T cells recognize antigen fragments and destroy specific target cells. Natural killer cells are lymphocytes that play an important role in tumor surveillance, natural resistance, hematopoiesis, adaptive immunity, and graft-versus-host reactions.

Soluble Mediators of the Immune System

Soluble mediators are responsible for cell-to-cell communication:

- *Antibodies* are serum glycoprotiens that have specificity to particular antigens (e.g., IgG is the major antibody produced in a secondary immune response).
- *Cytokines* are substances produced by immune cells that mediate the activity of other cells.
- *Serum proteins* control inflammation by, first, binding and coating bacteria, thereby promoting phagocytosis; and, second, increasing vascularity at the site, which increases capillary permeability, leading to cell lysis.
- *Prostaglandins* are major end products of arachidonic acid metabolism produced from inflammatory immune cells.

Mechanisms of Adaptive Immunity

Humoral Immune Response

Humoral immune responses act in defense against bacteria, viruses, and certain hypersensitivity reactions. The main mechanism involves the binding of antibodies to antigens. Antigens can stimulate B cells to become antibody-producing plasma cells. When an antibody binds to a particular antigen, an immune complex is formed. The major roles of antibodies are to

- neutralize bacterial and viral toxins,
- coat bacteria, rendering it recognizable as foreign by phagocytes, and
- activate complement, which forms a protein complex and promotes destruction by phagocytes.

Cell-Mediated Immune Response
The T cells are responsible for cell-mediated immunity. Maturation and proliferation of T cells take place in the thymus. When T cells encounter a recognizable antigen in the body, they proliferate. Subpopulations of T cells are produced against the same antigen but may have different functions, including cytotoxicity, memory, helper, or suppressor functions.

Delayed-Type Hypersensitivity
T cells mediate delayed-type hypersensitivity reactions. Inflammatory CD4 cells recognize receptors on major histocompatibility complexes, usually in response to a previously responded pathogen. An example of this process is the tuberculin skin test.

Cell-Mediated Cytotoxicity
Cell-mediated cytotoxicity is the recognition and lysis of target cells. On contact with the target cell (cancer cell or virus) the effector cell (NK cell or T cell) releases perforin, a protein substance that causes the formation of pores on the target cell membrane, leading to an influx of water, electrolytes, and enzymes, which causes the target cell to burst. Protectin, a protective protein, protects the effector cell during this process. Individuals with metastatic cancer have lower NK function compared with those with earlier stages of malignancy, which supports the importance of NK function in the survival of individuals with cancer.

Tissue Destruction from Immune Responses

Neutrophils and macrophages produce toxins during inflammation and phagocytosis, which may lead to damage of healthy cells. Ingestion of antioxidants may help to repair these normal cells.

Factors Affecting Immune Responses

The neuroendocrine and immune systems are thought to play a significant role in mediating stress and in the relationship between the stress response and disease. Numerous factors enhance or suppress the immune function:

- Cognitive–behavioral and other stress-reducing interventions have been associated with improvements in immune function and survival in cancer patients.
- Advancing age is associated with decline of immune function, specifically T-cell deterioration.
- Female reproductive hormones may affect immune responses; specifically, increased levels of estrogen and progesterone have been found to have a negative effect on immune function.
- Protein calorie and zinc deficiencies are associated with suppressed cell-mediated immune mechanisms. Vitamins A, C, and E and selenium promote maintenance of healthy cells. Soy proteins also may affect immune function and cancer growth.
- Alcohol and other drugs may suppress NK cytotoxicity. Marijuana, caffeine, and smoking also affect immune function.
- Physical exercise has a positive effect on the immune system, specifically NK cytotoxicity.
- Growth hormone and prolactin are associated with enhanced immune function and are elevated during sleep.

Chapter 3

Carcinogenesis

Normally, the body's cells are held under rigid growth control. The control of this growth or cell division is maintained by oncogenes (growth promoters) and cancer-suppressor genes (growth inhibitors).

Carcinogenesis is the process by which these genes and cells lose their normal control mechanisms of growth and then proliferate out of control.

Stages of Carcinogenesis

Carcinogenesis involves three major steps: initiation, promotion, and progression.

1. *Initiation* indicates a primary change in the target produced by a carcinogen.
2. *Promotion* is the secondary effect of a promoter, which alone might not be able to induce a malignancy.
3. *Progression* is the process by which tumors go from bad to worse.

Distinction among the steps in carcinogenesis is blurred, and there may be many more steps than those listed. More than one type of initiating event is probably common. In some cases, initiators may act as their own promoters (a complete carcinogen). An initiator may be a complete carcinogen for one organ and an incomplete carcinogen for another organ.

Carcinogenesis can be classified as chemical, familial, physical, or viral. Carcinogenesis also can be classified as occupational, dietary, environmental, or lifestyle.

Chemical Carcinogenesis

There are few chemicals for which there is strong evidence of cancer causation in humans. Tobacco is directly identified as a carcinogen. Some industrial chemicals are known to cause cancer, such as benzene, 2-naphthylamine, vinyl chloride, and some metals. Only 4% of cancer deaths in the United States are due to occupational exposure. Chemotherapeutic agents are carcinogenic and are associated with subsequent development of cancer, especially leukemia and myeloproliferative syndromes.

Familial Carcinogenesis

Some genes, when inherited, increase the risk of cancer. Fifteen percent of human cancers may have an hereditary component. About 35 familial cancer syndromes have been identified and include retinoblastoma, Wilms' tumor, neurofibromatosis types 1 and 2, familial polyposis associated with colon cancer, syndromes of multiple endocrine neoplasias, von Hippel-Lindau syndrome, Fanconi's anemia, ataxia telangiectasia, Bloom syndrome, Li-Fraumeni syndrome, xeroderma pigmentosum, hereditary nonpolyposis colorectal cancer (HNPCC), and dysplastic nevus syndrome.

Breast cancer is estimated to have a familial component in about 13% of cases. The most well known familial genetic links are *BRCA1* in breast and ovarian cancer and *BRCA2* in breast cancer.

Physical Carcinogenesis

Physical carcinogens are agents that damage oncogenes and cancer-suppressor genes by physical means. Ultraviolet radiation from the sun induces cancers of the skin. Ionizing radiation, mostly from natural sources, is carcinogenic. Asbestos causes mesothelioma and bronchogenic cancers.

Viral Carcinogenesis

Evidence for viral etiology of cancer is strongest for

- hepatitis B virus (HBV) and hepatocellular carcinoma,
- human T-cell leukemia virus type 1 (HTLV-1) and T-cell lymphoma,
- Burkitt's lymphoma and Epstein-Barr virus (EBV), and
- herpes simplex virus type 2 (HSV-2) and human papillomavirus (HPV) in cervical carcinoma.

Bacterial Carcinogenesis

A carcinogenesis relationship has been discovered between *Helicobacter pylori* and the mucosa-associated lymphoid tissue (MALT) lymphoma of the gastric mucosa. Chronic *H. pylori* gastritis is also associated with gastric adenocarcinoma.

Controversies in Carcinogenesis

Several scientific controversies in the field of carcinogenesis exist for which there is no certain answer. These include the relationship between estrogens (contraceptives, estrogen replacement) and breast cancer, involuntary (passive) smoking and lung cancer, environmental (lifestyle) and AIDS, and diet and cancer.

Chapter 4
••••••••••••

Cancer Control and Epidemiology

Cancer epidemiology examines the frequency of cancer in populations, the role of risk factors that contribute to cancer, and the interrelationships between host and environment.

Environmental Factors Associated with Cancer Causation

Tobacco
Tobacco use is the most important known cause of cancer and causes about 30% of cancer deaths. Cigarette smoking causes 90% of lung cancers. The use of chewing tobacco and snuff is increasing among male youth.

Diet
Diet has been proposed as a contributing factor in 20% to 70% of cancer deaths. It is a modifiable risk factor. Current issues regarding diet and cancer are

- high fat intake and risk of colon cancer,
- the protective effect of fiber and calcium intake against colon cancer,
- high fat intake and risk of breast cancer, and
- the protective effect of fruits and vegetables.

Alcohol
The use of alcohol accounts for 3% of cancer deaths. Alcohol is causally linked with cancers of the oral cavity, pharynx, larynx, esophagus, and liver, and may be linked to cancers of the breast and rectum. Additionally, alcohol appears to be synergistic with smoking.

Physical Activity
Increased physical activity is protective for colon cancer and precancerous colon polyps, and it may be protective for breast cancer.

Occupational Exposures
Approximately 4% to 9% of cancer deaths can be attributed to exposure to occupational carcinogens. The lung is the most commonly affected site. Some occupational carcinogens include asbestos, pesticides, benzene, benzidine, ether, cadmium compounds, vinyl chloride, and wood dusts.

Pollution
Air pollution may contribute to lung cancer deaths. An association between water pollution and cancer risk is unproved. The deterioration of the ozone layer may increase the risk for skin cancer.

Reproductive Factors and Sexual Behavior
Risk factors related to reproduction and sexual behavior have been identified only for cancers in women. They are listed in Table 4.1.

Table 4.1 Risk Factors Related to Reproduction and Sexual Behavior			
Risk factor	Breast	Cervical/ Endometrial	Ovarian
Early menopause	X	X	X
Late menopause	X	X	X
Nulliparity	X	X	X
Late first pregnancy (> 35 years old)	X		
Obesity	X*		X
Multiple sexual partners		X	

*Postmenopausal women only

Viruses

Viruses contribute to 15% to 20% of worldwide cancer incidence. Implicated viruses and cancer include those in Table 4.2.

Radiation

Approximately 20% of cancer deaths are due to radiation sources, excluding occupational exposures. Types of radiation are

- Ionizing (e.g., x-rays)
- Nonionizing (e.g., electrical power, radar, microwave sources)
- Ultraviolet (UV)

Drugs

Drugs associated with malignancies include the following:

- Alkylating agents: most closely linked with second malignancies
- Phenacetin: associated with cancers of the lower urinary tract
- Azathioprine: associated with increased incidence of lymphoma and squamous-cell skin cancer
- Cyclosporine: associated with risk of lymphoma

Table 4.2 Implicated Viruses and Cancers

Virus	Cancer
Hepatitis B virus (HBV)	Hepatocellular carcinoma
Human T-lymphotropic virus type 1 (HTLV-1)	Adult T-cell leukemia/ lymphoma
Epstein-Barr virus (EBV)	Burkitt's lymphoma
Human papillomavirus (HPV)	Cervical cancer
Helicobacter pylori	Gastric cancer
Schistosoma	Bladder cancer

- 8-Methoxypsoralen combined with UV radiation (used for treatment of psoriasis and vitiligo): associated with increased risk of squamous cell cancer of the skin

Exogenous Hormones

Exogenous hormones that influence an increased or decreased risk for cancer include the following:

- Diethylstilbestrol: associated with vaginal and cervical cancers in daughters of treated women
- Combined oral contraceptives: associated with decreased risk of endometrial and ovarian cancer
- Oral contraceptive use in young women: associated with increased risk of liver cancer
- Estrogen replacement therapy: shown to increase the risk of endometrial cancer in postmenopausal women

Host Characteristics Influencing Cancer Susceptibility

Age

Individuals over age 65 are 10 times more likely to develop cancer because of

- prolonged lifetime exposure to cancer-inducing agents and
- declining efficacy of the immune system.

Sex

The prostate is the leading site of cancer in men, followed by the lung and bronchus and colon/rectum. The leading site of cancer in women is the breast, followed by the lung and bronchus and colon/rectum.

Genetic Predisposition

Developments in molecular biology have increased the investigation of genetic predisposition to cancer. New gene markers are being identified. Investigations have revealed the following:

- Genetic predisposition is associated with certain types of cancer, such as familial polyposis.
- Cancer aggregates in some families are due to inherited susceptibility or to common environmental exposure.
- Two genes, BRCA1 and BRCA2, are associated with 5% of breast cancers.

Ethnicity and Race
Biologic and cultural factors cause differences in incidence and mortality.

Socioeconomic Factors
Socioeconomic status is not a cause of cancer but is a proxy measure for lifestyle characteristics that differ for cancer type. For example, cervical cancer is associated with a lower socioeconomic level, but it may be due to number of sexual partners or frequency of Pap smears. Socioeconomic status is now strongly associated with smoking prevalence and higher lung cancer rates, with low-income earners more likely to smoke cigarettes.

Cancer Control
Cancer control is the attempt to reduce cancer incidence, morbidity, and mortality through cancer prevention and research on interventions.

Screening
Screening refers to the detection of disease by the use of tests, examinations, or other procedures prior to the development of symptoms. Epidemiology is important in the development and evaluation of screening programs.

Barriers to Participation in Screening Programs
General barriers to participation in screening programs include cost, availability, time, discrimination, and patient characteristics. Lack of behavioral change by high-risk individuals and lack of monies appropriated by the government affect cancer control efforts.

Application to Nursing Practice

Epidemiologic data are used by nurses to

- identify high-risk patient populations,
- understand survival rates (calculation of the probability that an individual with a specific disease will be alive at a particular time after diagnosis [usually 5 years]), and
- develop and evaluate the effectiveness of a cancer prevention program.

Part II

Prevention, Detection, and Diagnosis

Chapter 5

Dynamics of Cancer Prevention

The focus of cancer treatment and cure by clinicians, researchers, and funding agencies is slowly beginning to shift to cancer prevention. Cancer prevention is a component of cancer control.

Definitions of Cancer Prevention

The traditional definitions of *cancer prevention* (primary, secondary, tertiary), which encompass the health continuum, do not reflect the evolving science of cancer prevention. Currently, primary prevention relates to initiation, secondary prevention to promotion, and tertiary prevention to progression. Examples are as follows:

- *Primary prevention*: avoidance of exposure to carcinogens and tobacco use, changes in diet, and administration of chemopreventive agents to healthy individuals
- *Secondary prevention*: prevention of promotion by smoking cessation, changes in diet, and use of chemopreventive agents to act on promotion
- *Tertiary prevention*: arresting, removing, or reversing a premalignant lesion to prevent recurrence or progression

Modern Approaches to Cancer Prevention

Education and Knowledge

Cancer prevention education focuses on changing lifestyle behaviors. Educational efforts need to persuade people to adopt preventive behaviors and to put acquired knowledge into practice.

Regulation

Much of the regulations related to cancer prevention are a result of public demand. Examples of regulation are

- state laws that ban the sale of cigarettes to young people and
- excise taxes on alcohol products, to increase their cost, thereby reducing their accessibility.

Host Modification

Host modification is the alteration of the body's internal environment to prevent initiation or progression of cancer. The principal methods are immunization and chemoprevention.

- *Immunization:* Approaches to cancer vaccines are being explored and cancer vaccine trials are under way.
- *Chemoprevention:* The most promising form of host modification is chemoprevention, or the use of nutrients (e.g., betacarotene, vitamins, selenium) or pharmacological agents (e.g., tamoxifen, synthetic retinoids, NSAIDs), to inhibit or reverse the process of carcinogenesis. Chemopreventive agents enhance the inactivation of carcinogens, modify the expression of oncogenes, or interfere with cell proliferation.

Chemoprevention Research

The National Cancer Institute (NCI) established the chemoprevention research program to look at chemoprevention and diet and nutrition. Numerous phase I and phase II trials are under way. High-priority trials include the following:

- Study of tamoxifen and raloxifine in postmenopausal women 35 years or older who are at increased risk of developing cancer
- Prostate cancer prevention trial testing the ability of finasteride to prevent prostate cancer in healthy men aged 55 and older

PART II

Chapter 6
....

Counseling on Genetic Risk for Cancer

Risk assessment is an important component of cancer prevention. The ability to identify individuals who are at increased risk for developing cancer will allow screening programs and prevention strategies to be targeted to those individuals most in need.

Cancer Risk Assessment
The goals of risk assessment are to

- understand an individual's perception related to risk for developing cancer,
- provide information regarding that risk,
- outline recommendations for prevention, and
- offer psychosocial support so that an individual may better cope with risk-related information and adhere to recommendations for prevention and screening.

A review of the individual's medical and lifestyle history will provide information related to risk for developing cancer. A review of family history will help determine the risk of a hereditary cancer syndrome.

Hereditary Cancer Syndromes
The genes associated with hereditary cancer are rapidly being identified. However, only 5% to 10% of cancers are due to inheritance of a gene. The most common hereditary cancer syndromes are

- ataxia telangiectasia,
- breast/ovarian cancer,
- hereditary nonpolyposis colorectal cancer (HNPCC),

- familial adenomatous polyposis (FAP),
- Li-Fraumeni syndrome,
- malignant melanoma,
- multiple endocrine neoplasia (MEN) types 1 and 2, and
- retinoblastoma.

Several common characteristics seen in families with a hereditary cancer syndrome include

- occurrence of multiple cases of cancer within a single lineage (e.g., maternal side or paternal side),
- diagnosis of cancer at an earlier age than that seen in the general population,
- occurrence of multiple cancers in one person,
- the presence of rare tumors,
- cancer in paired organs, and
- nonmalignant manifestations of an hereditary cancer syndrome.

Individuals with these characteristics should be referred for intensive cancer genetic counseling.

Hereditary Breast and Ovarian Cancer Syndromes

Syndromes of breast cancer susceptibility are linked to mutations in BRCA1 and BRCA2. Ovarian cancer is also seen in women carrying mutations in these two genes.

Hereditary Colon Cancers

Cancer susceptibility syndromes account for 5% of colorectal cancers. The most common syndrome is hereditary nonpolyposis colorectal cancer (HNPCC). Familial adenomatous polyposis (FAP) is less frequent.

Genetic Risk Counseling

Genetic counseling involves risk assessment and information gathering, evaluation and analysis of data, communication of genetic and risk information (e.g., limitations of genetic tests, benefits, costs, risk, and meaning of results), supportive counseling, and follow-up counseling. Genetic testing should be conducted only in conjunction with genetic counseling. A new role for oncology nurses will be to participate in the provision of cancer genetic risk counseling.

Problems and Issues Related to Genetic Testing

Setting for Testing
Many contend that genetic testing should be done only in a research setting, because many unanswered questions remain. When to test for genes is another issue.

Informed Consent
Adequate information must be provided for individuals to give written informed consent.

Accuracy of Test and Interpretation of Results
The counselor must review how the test is performed, the type of test, the sensitivity and specificity of the test, who in the family is the best person to test, potential answers that may be obtained, and the meaning of each answer.

Psychosocial Issues
Assessing the psychological impact of test results is important. The confidentiality of results remains an area of question and concern. Serious consideration must be given to how test results are documented, communicated, and managed to ensure confidentiality.

Management of Risk
Measures to manage risk for those carrying a mutation are important. Management options fall into three categories:

1. *Chemoprevention* (e.g., nonsteroidal antiin-flammatory drugs for prevention of colorec-

tal cancer, or tamoxifen for prevention of breast cancer)
2. *Prophylactic surgery* (e.g., prophylactic mastectomy)
3. *Screening and detection* at frequent intervals and at an earlier patient age

Chapter 7

Diagnostic Evaluation, Classification, and Staging

Diagnostic Evaluation

The etiology of most cancers is unknown, and cancer prevention measures are complicated by economic, behavioral, social, and cultural factors. The key to survival is early detection. The worst prognosis can be expected in persons who delay seeking medical evaluation at the onset of their symptoms.

Factors Affecting the Diagnostic Approach

The major goals of the diagnostic evaluation are to determine

- tissue type,
- primary site of the malignancy,
- extent of disease, and
- risk of recurrence.

The seven warning signals of cancer are

C: Change in bowel or bladder habits,

A: A sore that does not heal,

U: Unusual bleeding or discharge,

T: Thickening or a lump in a breast or elsewhere,

I: Indigestion or difficulty in swallowing,

O: Obvious change in wart or mole, and

N: Nagging cough or hoarseness.

Nursing Implications

Nurses may promote the early detection and diagnosis of cancer by

- serving as role models by incorporating early

detection practices in their own personal health care,

- increasing public awareness through communication and education,
- teaching patients about the importance of early detection,
- designing community education programs that target high-risk clients,
- performing early-detection examinations (pelvic examinations, Papanicolaou tests, and testicular and breast examinations),
- displaying posters and American Cancer Society pamphlets of cancer's warning signals, and
- providing information and support to reduce the stress of going through a diagnostic evaluation for a suspected malignancy.

Laboratory Techniques

Laboratory studies are performed to help confirm a clinical diagnosis and to monitor the patient's response to treatment. The accuracy of a particular laboratory procedure is reported in terms of sensitivity or specificity:

- *Sensitivity*: the percentage of people with cancer who will have an abnormal test result (true positive). Test results of people with cancer that are negative (normal) are false-negative.
- *Specificity*: the percentage of people without cancer who will have negative (normal) test results, known as true-negative. Test results of people who are free of disease and show positive (abnormal) results are false-positive.
- A clinically useful test will detect a malignant abnormality early in its development (sensitivity) and exclude nonmalignant sources for the abnormality (specificity).

Biochemical analysis of blood and urine identifies chemical and hematological values. Tumor markers are proteins, antigens, or genes that are tumor derived or tumor associated. An increase or decrease can indicate tumor response, locate the tumor's origin, or determine recurrence. The most commonly used tumor markers are listed in Table 7.1.

Diagnostic and prognostic information in a variety of cancers has improved due to technological advances in radioimmunoassay and flow cytometry.

Tumor Imaging

Many diagnostic procedures can determine the presence of a tumor mass, localize the mass for biopsy, and stage the extent of disease:

- Radiological techniques include chest x-ray, mammogram, tomography, and computerized tomography.
- Nuclear medicine techniques include positron emission tomography (PET), gallium scans, bone scans, and radiolabeled monoclonal antibodies.

Table 7.1 Common Tumor Markers	
Tumor Marker	Associated Malignancy (Elevated)
Carcinoembryonic antigen (CEA)	Colorectal, stomach, pancreas, lung, and breast cancer
Alpha-fetoprotein (AFP)	Testicular, hepatocellular, colon, lung, and stomach cancer
Human chorionic gonadotropin beta-subunit (B-HCG)	Choriocarcinoma, germ-cell tumors of testicle and ovary
Prostate-specific antigen (PSA)	Prostate cancer
Cancer antigen 125 (CA 125)	Ovary, pancreas, breast, colon, lung, and liver cancer
Cancer antigen 19-9 (CA 19-9)	Pancreas, colon, and gastric cancer
Cancer antigen 15-3 (CA 15-3)	Breast cancer
Cancer antigen 27.29 (CA 27.29)	Breast cancer
Cancer antigen 72-4 (CA 72-4)	Gastric cancer

- Ultrasonography measures reflecting echoes of sound waves of specific tissues.
- Magnetic resonance imaging creates sectional images of the body without exposure to ionizing radiation.

Invasive Diagnostic Techniques

The numerous invasive techniques are summarized as follows:

- *Endoscopy* provides a direct view by insertion of an endoscope into a body cavity or opening and permits visual inspection, tissue biopsy, cytologic aspiration, staging of disease, and excision for pathology.
- *Needle biopsy* provides histological or cytological proof of malignancy.
  - Fine-needle aspiration (FNA) provides cytological and microhistological information.
  - Stereotactic localization uses CT or MRI to localize a lesion.
  - Core needle biopsy removes more than does FNA.
- *Surgical biopsy*
- *Incisional biopsy* removes a portion of the mass for pathological examination.
- *Excisional biopsy* removes the entire mass.
- *Laparoscopy* is used for the detection, staging, and treatment of cancer (lymphoma, gastrointestinal, urological, and gynecological).

Classification and Nomenclature

Benign and Malignant Tumor Characteristics

The following features distinguish between a benign and malignant tumor.

Characteristics of a benign tumor:

- Slow-growing, often encapsulated
- Does not invade normal tissue
- Does not metastasize

- Cells are uniform, well-differentiated and resemble the tissue of origin.

Characteristics of a malignant tumor:

- High mitotic rate
- Rapid growth
- Local tissue invasion
- Rare encapsulation
- Metastasis to distant sites
- Anaplastic and poorly differentiated tumor cells

Tumor Classification System

Tumors are classified by biological behavior and tissue of origin:

- Carcinoma: malignant tumor of epithelial tissues
- Sarcoma: malignant tumor of the connective tissues
- Blastoma: malignant tumor of embryonic development
- Lymphoma, melanoma, and hepatoma: malignant tumors with -*oma* suffix
- Hodgkin's disease, Ewing's sarcoma, and Wilms' tumor: malignancies named after the person who described them
- Hematopoietic malignancies: classified by cell type and are acute or chronic in nature

Staging and Grading Classifications

The goals of staging

- determine extent of disease
- provide information for treatment planning
- give prognostic information
- assist in treatment evaluation
- facilitate exchange of information and compare statistics
- stratify individuals for clinical trial accrual

The TNM classification system describes the anatomical extent of disease for solid tumors.

TNM definitions:

- **T**: the primary tumor is evaluated on the basis of depth of invasion, surface spread, and tumor size
- **N**: the absence or presence and extent of regional lymph node metastasis with attention to the size and location of the nodes
- **M**: the absence or presence of distant metastasis

TNM classifications:

- cTNM: clinical assessment
- pTNM: pathological or postsurgical assessment
- rTNM: assessment at the time of retreatment following recurrence
- aTNM: assessment at the time of death/ autopsy

PART II

Patient Performance Classification

The evaluation of patient performance helps to determine the patient's functional status and eligibility for treatment. The most frequently used scales are:

- Karnofsky scale: 0% to 100%, where 100% is normal activity
- ECOG scale: 4–0, where 0 is normal activity
- WHO scale: 4–0, where 0 is normal activity

Grading

Grading is a method of classification based on histopathological characteristics of the tissue:

- GX: grade cannot be assessed
- G1: well-differentiated
- G2: moderately well-differentiated
- G3: poorly differentiated
- G4: undifferentiated

Part III

Treatment

Chapter 8

Principles of Treatment Planning and Clinical Research

Factors Involved in Treatment Planning

Treatment Goals

Treatment of cancer is intended to achieve one of three outcomes:

1. Cure

2. Control and prolongation of life

3. Palliation of symptoms

However, goals can overlap. An individual may undergo treatment for cure and then, years later, require additional therapy for recurrent disease or palliation. A determination of whether to treat for cure is one of the most critical treatment decisions. The basic principle is to cure, if possible, with minimal structural and functional impairment.

Treatment Planning Variables

Numerous factors that influence cancer treatment choices must be considered when setting a goal and selecting the most appropriate treatment plan:

- *Tumor factors:* Histology and stage are key factors in predicting tumor aggressiveness. Staging provides the best predictor of potential success. However, anatomical location may limit options.

- *Treatment factors:* Prior cancer treatment, if any, is evaluated. The availability and effectiveness of treatment modalities must be reviewed carefully, and enrollment in a clinical trial may be best. Treatment benefit is measured by the response of the tumor:

- Complete response is disappearance of all signs of cancer for two or more evaluations separated by 4 weeks.
- Partial response refers to at least a 50% reduction in size of tumor mass for 4 or more weeks.

The interaction of potential treatments and overlapping side effects need to be considered.

- *Patient factors:* Concomitant disease or illness requires adjustment of the treatment plan. Performance status predicts tolerance. Patient preference regarding aggressiveness of treatment will vary. Age is an important factor if growth is still occurring or if fertility may be affected by treatment.

Treatment Planning Throughout the Continuum

Treatment Aimed at Cure or Complete Response

Curative therapy is often undertaken for localized or early-stage disease, but some advanced-stage cancers can be cured (e.g., testicular cancer, Hodgkin's disease, osteogenic carcinoma).

Treatment for cure must be aggressive, and the first treatment is the best and often only opportunity for cure. Treatment for cure options include the following:

- Surgery is often the primary approach
- Adjuvant therapy for localized disease (e.g., radiation or chemotherapy)
  - Can eliminate potential micrometastases
  - Can enable a less radical surgery
- Primary or neoadjuvant therapy is chemotherapy or radiation sequenced before surgery
- Chemotherapy or radiation therapy alone or in combination

Treatment for Advanced or Recurrent Disease
The treatment goal is to prolong survival and possibly provide cure. Some patients may have long symptom-free periods. Chemotherapy, radiation therapy, and surgery are used to control locally advanced disease. Surgery can be used to debulk the tumor mass and thus enhance the effect of chemotherapy or radiation therapy.

Palliative Treatment
Palliative treatment is used when prolonging life is no longer an option. Treatment may involve any single or combined modality. Palliative treatment should minimize cost, inconvenience, discomfort, and risks.

Principles of Clinical Research
Clinical trials are highly controlled research experiments that require careful planning and rigorous conduct. Cooperative research groups, cancer centers, and pharmaceutical companies sponsor research studies. The research study is detailed in a written protocol that defines the patient characteristics for inclusion or exclusion, the treatment to be given, and the evaluation methods to be used.

Clinical Trials of New Chemotherapeutic Agents
The clinical evaluation of new agents is conducted in 4 phases.

- *Phase I trials*: establish the maximum tolerated dose of the drug (not effectiveness). Eligibility for a trial is broad. Patients must have proven disease for which no effective treatment plan exists. Dose escalation is a part of this phase.
- *Phase II trials*: prove the drug's effectiveness against specific tumors and determine whether the drug should undergo further evaluation. Careful patient selection occurs to ensure

meaningful results. The usual measure of a drug's effectiveness is tumor response, whether total or partial.

- *Phase III trials*: A new treatment is compared with standard therapy. A drug may be tested as a single agent or as part of combination therapy. Phase III trials require hundreds of participants in order to have meaningful results. The study is usually a prospective, randomized trial.
- *Phase IV trials*: Following Food and Drug Administration approval, these postmarketing studies are not required but can be used to obtain new information about any risks or side effects not previously identified.

Clinical Trials in Surgical Oncology
Most aspects of these trials are similar to those of chemotherapy trials. Because the success of a new surgical technique may be dependent on the surgeon's skills, the evaluation of surgical approaches is difficult. Standard approaches and techniques are important to put in place.

Clinical Trials in Radiation Oncology
Radiation is known to be effective in cancer treatment, so trials concentrate on comparing delivery methods, schedules, and different combinations of therapy. Both initial tumor response and locoregional control are evaluated.

Issues in Oncology Clinical Trials
In the United States, the approval process is rigorous. Safeguards are in place to avoid harm or undue risk:

- Exclusion criteria restrict the eligibility of persons who wish to enter trials, to assure meaningful conclusions.
- Patients may feel that entering a clinical trial offers their best hope for cure, and many become aggressive in their search for a trial to

PART III

enter. Forthright discussions about eligibility, prognosis, and outcome, combined with hope, are needed.

- Randomized trials can create conflict for clinicians between their roles as clinician and their role as researcher. Individual experience may bias a clinician toward a standard approach, yet the potential for a new approach must also be explored.

Chapter 9

Surgical Therapy

Surgery is the most frequently used cancer therapy. It offers the greatest hope for cure. Surgery is used alone or in combination with other cancer therapies. Using combinations of surgery, chemotherapy, radiotherapy, and biotherapy has significantly lengthened disease-free intervals, and survival advantages have been realized.

Surgery can be used for

- cancer prevention,
- diagnosis,
- definitive treatment,
- rehabilitation, and
- palliation.

PART III

Factors Influencing Surgical Oncology

About 75% of surgical procedures performed in the United States occur within an ambulatory setting. Educating the patient and family in patient self-care following surgery is a significant challenge to health care workers.

Advances in surgical technology have led to less invasive surgical procedures, resulting in fewer surgical risks, less pain, and a less extensive recovery period. Lasers, laparoscopes, and endoscopes are a few of the technologies used.

Economic forces and managed care have precipitated aggressive measures to reduce lengthy and costly hospital stays.

Factors Influencing Treatment Decisions

Tumor Cell Kinetics

Knowledge of tumor cell kinetics has helped clinicians identify tumors that are best treated with surgery. The goal is to eradicate the tumor with the least amount of disruption to normal tissue. Decisions about the extent of surgical resection are guided by characteristics of tumor cells:

- *Growth rate*: Slow-growing tumors lend themselves best to surgical treatment because they are more likely to be confined locally.
- *Invasiveness*: A surgical procedure intended to be curative must include resection of the entire tumor mass and a margin of safety that includes normal tissue surrounding the tumor. Less radical procedures are indicated with invasive disease, for which radical surgery has not been proved to enhance results.
- *Metastatic potential*: The initial surgical procedure has a better chance of success than any subsequent surgery performed for recurrence. Knowledge of metastatic patterns of individual tumors is crucial for planning the most effective therapy. Some tumors metastasize late or not at all and may respond well to aggressive primary surgical resection. For tumors known to metastasize early, surgery may not be appropriate. Surgery may be used to remove a tumor mass either in preparation for adjuvant systemic therapy or after chemotherapy to resect any remaining disease.

Tumor Location
The location and extent of tumor determine the structural and functional changes after surgery. Superficial and encapsulated tumors are more easily resected than are those embedded in inaccessible or delicate tissues or those that have invaded tissues in multiple directions.

Physical Status
Preoperative assessment is intended to identify factors that may increase the risk of surgical morbidity and mortality. The patient's rehabilitation potential is assessed before surgery.

Quality of Life

The goal of surgical therapy varies with the stage of disease. Selection of treatment approach takes into consideration the quality of the individual's life when treatment is complete.

Preventing Cancer Using Surgical Procedures

Surgery may remove nonvital benign tissue that predisposes individuals to a higher risk of cancer, such as the prophylactic removal of the breast in women with a high risk of breast cancer. Removal of precancerous polyps is commonly done as a measure to prevent colon cancer.

Diagnosing Cancer Using Surgical Techniques

Only positive biopsy findings are definitive in a diagnosis of cancer. The biopsy specimen should contain both normal cells and tumor cells for comparison. A limitation is the possibility that the tumor will be missed.

There are three types of surgical biopsies:

1. Excisional biopsy is performed on small, accessible tumors to remove the entire mass and little or no margin of surrounding normal tissues.
2. Incisional biopsy is used to diagnose large tumors that require major surgery for complete removal.
3. Endoscopy is used for the diagnosis of tumors in accessible lumen.

Staging Cancer Using Surgical Procedures

Exploratory surgical procedures are important in defining the extent of tumor involvement. Determining the stage of disease is important in the selection of therapy.

Surgery for Treatment of Cancer

Surgery Aimed at Cure

The surgical approach for cure has changed from a "more is better" philosophy to consideration of tissue and functional preservation. The type of surgical procedure selected depends on specific tumor-cell characteristics and site of involvement.

Adjuvant or combination therapy including radiotherapy or chemotherapy may be used to improve cure rates and survival.

Surgery may be used to resect a metastatic lesion if the primary tumor is believed to be eradicated and the metastatic site is solitary.

Surgery Aimed at Palliation

Surgery can be used for palliation of debilitating manifestations of cancer, such as pain and obstruction. Palliative therapy is aimed at controlling cancer and improving quality of life.

Surgery for Rehabilitation

Rehabilitative surgery is used for cosmetic reasons or to restore function after surgery, such as breast reconstruction, head and neck reconstruction, and skin grafting. The goal is to improve quality of life.

Special Considerations for Nursing Care

More surgical procedures are now done on an ambulatory basis. Ambulatory surgery presents challenges for nurses to minimize postoperative complications and maximize patient support and education. Particularly challenging is the patient with concomitant diseases receiving aggressive treatment for cancer.

Surgical Setting and Length of Stay

The greatest challenge concerning the short length of stay for surgical procedures is to ensure that adequate information is given to patients and families, so that they are well educated in regard to the procedure and the care afterward.

General Surgical Care and Oncological Emergencies

In addition to the typical surgical complications, cancer patients may experience a complex set of responses precipitated by concomitant therapies or the underlying disease process itself. These can include acute respiratory distress syndrome (ARDS), aspiration pneumonia, infection, bleeding, poor wound healing, and stomatitis. Blood product administration, pain control, nutritional support, and hemostasis are common surgical challenges.

Autologous Blood Donation

Patients may donate one or more units of their own blood to bank before surgery (autologous blood donation). Autologous donation may be done 42 days to 72 hours before surgery.

Anxiety and Pain Control

Teaching about pain control begins preoperatively and includes expectations of pain and relief measures, use of rating scales to measure pain, and nonpharmacological methods to decrease pain and anxiety.

Nutritional Support

The nutritionally debilitated person with cancer is a poor surgical risk. Before surgery, protein calorie malnutrition should be reversed. Patients may receive aggressive preoperative nutritional support to improve nutritional status.

Hemostasis

The person with cancer is highly susceptible to postoperative thrombophlebitis. Early postoperative ambulation is instituted.

Combination Therapy

Synergistic and augmented effects of combined therapies can produce postoperative reactions and complications that may be difficult to manage. Radiotherapy and chemotherapy can compromise wound healing and may increase postoperative complications.

Chapter 10
• • • • • • • • • • • • •

Radiation Therapy

PART I. PRINCIPLES OF RADIATION THERAPY

Radiation therapy may be used as the sole treatment for cancer or in combination with surgery or chemotherapy or immunotherapy.

Goals of Treatment
The goal of radiation therapy may be to
- cure (e.g., skin cancer, carcinoma of cervix, Hodgkin's disease, or seminoma),
- control (e.g., breast cancer, soft-tissue sarcomas, or lung cancer), or
- palliate (e.g., relieving pain, preventing pathological fractures, relieving spinal cord compression).

Radiobiology
The biological effects of radiation are a sequence of events that follows the absorption of energy from ionizing radiation and the body's attempt to compensate for the assault.

Cellular Response to Radiation
Target theory would indicate that the radiation effect may be direct or indirect.

- A *direct hit* occurs when any key molecule within the cell (DNA or RNA) is damaged and leads to mutation and altered cell function or cell death. Direct hits produce the most effective radiation result.
- An *indirect hit* occurs when ionization takes place in the medium (mostly water) surrounding molecular structures in the cell. An indirect hit results in intracellular free radicals that trigger chemical reactions and produce com-

pounds that are toxic to the cell. Indirect hits are more likely to occur than direct hits.

Radiosensitivity of cells is

- directly proportional to cellular reproductive activity (radiation most effective during mitosis) and
- inversely proportional to cellular degree of differentiation (the more differentiated, the less sensitive to radiation).

Biologic factors that directly affect response to radiation include the following:

- Oxygen effect: Oxygen modifies the dose of radiation needed to produce biologic damage. Well-oxygenated tumors have a greater response to radiation.
- Dose rate: Dose rate refers to the rate at which a given dose is delivered by a treatment machine.
- Radiosensitivity: Ionizing radiation is most effective on cells that are undifferentiated and undergoing active mitosis.
- Fractionation: Fractionation involves dividing the total dose of radiation into a number of equal fractions.

Remembering the Four R's of radiobiology is a common way to consider how cells respond to radiation:

- *Repair:* Repair of sublethal damage to normal cells can occur between daily-dose fractions of radiation.
- *Redistribution:* Redistribution of cell age within the cell cycle as a result of daily radiation makes cells more radiosensitive.
- *Repopulation:* Repopulation of normal tissues takes place during a multifraction radiation treatment course.
- *Reoxygenation:* Tumor cells are characteristically normal to hypoxic, and fractionation allows time for the tumor to reoxygenate.

Radiobiology of Brachytherapy

Brachytherapy, the use of implanted or injected radioactive sources, capitalizes on continuous rather than fractionated approaches.

- *Low-dose rate brachytherapy* delivers a continuous dose of radiation for as long as the radioactive source remains in place within the patient. It is commonly used for gynecological and head and neck cancers.

- *High-dose rate brachytherapy* delivers more than 1200 cGy per hour as single, repeated fractions.

Radiolabeled Antibody Therapy

Radiolabled antibody therapy involves attachment of a radioactive substance to a tumor-specific antibody. The circulating antibody is taken up by the targeted organ, thereby delivering the radiation directly to the tumor site. The major limitation is the rapid clearance of the antibody, thus limiting the radiation effect.

Chemical and Thermal Modifiers of Radiation

Radiosensitizers and Radioprotectors

Certain agents and drugs can enhance or moderate the effect of radiation:

- *Radiosensitizers* increase the radiosensitivity of tumor cells; thus, radiation achieves greater cell kill by preventing repair of cellular radiation damage. Side effects include neurotoxicity; CNS symptoms of somnolence, confusion, and transient coma; and dose-related nausea and vomiting. Results with radiosensitizers are disappointing because of dose-limiting toxicity and lack of significant efficacy.

- *Radioprotectors* can protect oxygenated cells but have limited effect on hypoxic cells. These agents increase the therapeutic ratio by promoting repair of irradiated normal tissues.

PART II. TREATMENT PLANNING AND DELIVERY

Treatment Planning and Simulation Process

Treatment recommendations are based on potential for disease response and risk of acute and long-term toxicity. Treatment planning is a detailed and precise process to identify tumor type, size, and location.

Initial Consultation

Initial consultation includes a thorough history, physical examination, diagnostic work-up, discussion of treatment options, and informed consent.

Simulation

Simulation is used to define the tumor area to be treated. Simulation takes about 1 to 2 hours. The simulation process can be anxiety producing, so education and preparation are essential.

The process involves highly accurate measurements of patient characteristics to provide for differences in dose distribution, such as body contour, outline and depth of internal structures, and location and size of target.

A simulator is a specialized x-ray machine that can duplicate the geometry and mechanics of radiation treatment machines. Blocks are made to protect normal tissue from radiation where possible. Tattoos or skin markings are placed to guide replicating the treatment site.

Treatment Plan

The medical physicist and dosimetrist determine effective distribution of radiation. Specific planning computers aid the plan development and verification. Details of the treatment, such as beam angle, beam time, compensators, and blocks, are all designed individually.

Delivery of Radiation: External Beam or Teletherapy

Patients need to know to expect large machines with a rotating head, a hard treatment couch or table with removable sections, and a large treatment room. Once the treatment starts, the patient is in the room alone but is always monitored. The types of machines and equipment include linear accelerators and orthovoltage units.

Linear Accelerator

The linear accelerator delivers high-energy radiation and is the most frequently used contemporary radiation unit. The energy range of these megavoltage machines is wide, typically 4 to 20 MeV.

Multileaf collimators are new and provide computerized, customized blocking that does not require the creation of lead blocks and molds to shape the radiation beam to the desired target.

Orthovoltage Unit

This x-ray machine operates in the 150- to 500-kV range and is useful for treating superficial lesions.

Patient Positioning and Immobilizing Techniques

Positioning and immobilization are critical components for achieving the maximum dose desired to the target. Several techniques are used:

- *Immobilization devices* keep the patient in a stationary position for daily treatment and minimize the potential for treatment errors. Devices include tape and straps, body supports, and body casts.

- *Positioning devices* such as neck rolls, foam wedges, head holders, and neck supports help hold patients in nontraditional positions. Tilt boards, slant boards, and belly boards are also used.

PART III

Treatment Techniques

- *Intensity-modulated therapy* is a new technology for delivering a precise dose of radiation to the target while sparing surrounding normal tissues. The beam intensity can be varied to precise levels within a target.
- *Stereotactic radiosurgery* delivers the entire desired dose in one intense treatment. It is used mostly for intracranial lesions. Multiple beams are simultaneously delivered to the patient, who is immobilized in a positioning device.

Delivery of Radiation Implant Therapy or Brachytherapy

Brachytherapy or implant therapy is treatment in which the radiation source is in direct contact with the tumor. Brachytherapy can involve temporary or permanent implants. It can be combined with teletherapy and used preoperatively and postoperatively.

The source is selected by the radiotherapist according to the site to be treated, the size of the lesion, and whether the implant is temporary or permanent. Sources of brachytherapy can be contained in a variety of forms:

- Wires
- Ribbons or tubes
- Needles
- Grains or seeds
- Capsules

Brachytherapy is used in treatment of head and neck lesions (needles, wire, and ribbons), intraabdominal and intrathoracic lesions (gold or iodine seeds), and prostate cancer (seeds).

Three major factors are considered in developing safety plans for working with brachytherapy:

1. *Time:* Exposure to radiation is directly proportional to time spent within a specific distance from the source.

2. *Distance:* The amount of radiation reaching a given area decreases as the distance increases.

3. *Shield:* A sheet of absorbing material is placed between the radiation source and the detector. Portable radiation shields are available. They are useful for doing tasks within a room, but not for direct care.

Patient education includes the following:

- Description of procedure
- Preparation for potential change in appearance (needle implants in facial area)
- Knowledge of anticipated pain or discomfort and measures available for relief
- Knowledge of potential short-term and long-term side effects and complications
- Restrictions on activity while radioactive sources are in place
- Visiting restrictions
- Radiation precautions observed by hospital personnel
- Preparation for isolation by planning suitable activities, such as reading, doing handiwork, and watching television

PART III. TOXICITIES AND MANAGEMENT

Tissue and Organ Response to Radiation

All cells and structures that lie within the path of the radiation beam are vulnerable to toxicities.

Acute Effects

Acute effects occur mostly in rapidly renewing tissues and are seen in hours to days. Acute effects are site-specific, vary with each patient, and are usually short-term and resolve after the completion of therapy.

Subacute Effects
Subacute effects are clinically evident in a few weeks to months of completing radiation therapy.

Late Effects
The extent and degree of late effects depends on the site and total radiation dose. These effects are generally long lasting and do not resolve easily.

Management of Toxicities

Skin Reactions
The skin is irradiated when any site within the body is treated. Skin of the exit portal also may be affected. Skin reactions may be greater in skin in warm, moist areas, such as the groin, gluteal fold, axilla, and under the breast.

Acute reactions may occur within 2 to 3 weeks after the start of therapy.

- Skin reactions may range from erythema to dry or moist desquamation.
- Healing may be slow but is usually complete, leaving minimal residual damage, except for a change in pigmentation.

Chronic skin effects may occur months or years after therapy.

- Reactions may include fibrosis, ulceration, tissue necrosis, and hyperpigmentation.
- Skin cancer may occur after high doses but is uncommon with modern equipment.

Care of a skin reaction varies according to the severity of the reaction.

- Handling the skin gently is the most important approach.
- Goals generally include patient comfort, promotion of healing, and prevention of infection.

Radiation recall can occur in a previously irradiated site that exhibited mucositis or erythema.

- Recall occurs in response to systemic administration of certain chemotherapeutic agents
  several months to a year or more after radiation is received.
- A person can develop intraoral mucositis or a
  skin reaction in the exact pattern correspond-
  ing to a previously treated radiation portal.
- Treatment is supportive.

Fatigue
Fatigue is an expected side effect of radiation,
with 65% to 90% of patients reporting that
fatigue increases during therapy. Extra rest,
reduction in normal activity, and distraction are
among the measures used to treat fatigue. Pharmacologic and supportive therapies also may
be useful.

Myelosuppression
The bone marrow is highly radiosensitive and is
an important dose-limiting cell-renewal system
commonly affected by radiation. If large areas
containing bone marrow are in radiation fields,
then myelosuppression will be probable. Effects
include the following:

- Erythroblasts (red blood cell precursors) are
  damaged, causing anemia, but recovery is rapid
  and anemia is transient.
- Myeloblasts (white blood cell precursors) are
  suppressed at the same rate as erythroblasts,
  but rate of recovery is much slower.
- Megakaryocytes (platelet precursors) are
  affected 1 to 2 weeks after exposure and
  take the longest time to recover (2 to 6
  weeks).
- Recovery from severe myelosuppression can
  occur at least within 12 to 24 months.

To manage myelosuppression:
- Blood counts are done during radiotherapy
  weekly or two to three times weekly.

- Transfusions may be necessary for a patient with critically low blood counts.
- Radiation treatment may have to be adjusted or suspended.
- The patient should be observed for signs of bleeding, anemia, and infection.
- Teach the patient and family how to detect the early signs of myelosuppression.

Brain

Brain, spinal cord, and peripheral nerves are relatively radioresistant; damage relates to vascular insufficiency. Higher doses may produce transient symptoms in the central nervous system (CNS). The following toxicities can occur:

Alopecia and Scalp Erythema

- Due to the high mitotic rate of hair follicles, alopecia starts within 2 to 3 weeks of the start of therapy. Hair usually regrows with doses less than 6000 cGy.
- Alopecia follows a typical pattern. First the patient notices excessive amounts of hair in a brush or comb, followed by gradual thinning of the hair; this continues for about 2 or 3 weeks.
- Care of hair and scalp during radiation treatment:
  - Gentle brushing or combing
  - Infrequent shampooing
  - Permanent waves and hair coloring are contraindicated
  - The top of the patient's head should be protected from sunburn (e.g., wearing a cap).

Ear Symptoms

- If the ear is in the treatment field, the auditory canal can become irritated, sore, and pruritic.
- Cortisone ear drops and protective coverings can reduce the pain.

Cerebral Edema

- Increased intracranial pressure may be exacerbated by radiation to the brain.
- Corticosteroids are given to reduce edema.
- Teach the patient about side effects, tapering regimens, and signs of increasing pressure, such as headache, nausea, weakness, or mental changes.

Nausea and Vomiting

- Symptoms are short-lived and well controlled with antiemetics.
- Managing cerebral edema is critical to alleviating nausea and vomiting.

Somnolence Syndrome

- Somnolence syndrome occurs more often in children than in adults.
- Symptoms include excessive sleepiness and fatigue, anorexia, and mild headache.
- Treatment is supportive until the syndrome runs its course.

Head and Neck

Patients with tumors of the head and neck tend to have poor nutrition and poor oral hygiene. Numerous toxicities can occur.

Stomatitis

- The epithelial cells of the mucous membranes are highly radiosensitive. Reactions range from erythema to painful ulceration.
- Management
  - Practice excellent oral hygiene.
  - Avoid irritants, such as alcohol, tobacco, spicy or acidic foods, very hot or very cold foods and drinks, and commercial mouthwash products.
  - Swish and swallow as often as every 3 to 4 hours, and especially before bed, with a solution of 1 ounce of diphenhydramine hy-

PART III

drochloride (Benadryl), 1 ounce of liquid antacid, and 1 ounce of viscous lidocaine.

- Do not dislodge plaquelike formations of mucositis.

Xerostomia

- The major salivary glands are highly radiosensitive.
- An approximate 50% reduction in saliva production can occur after the first week of therapy. The remaining saliva can become very thick and ropy.
- Management strategies
  - Frequent sips of water
  - Frequent mouth care provides relief from thick and viscous saliva.
  - When inflammation has subsided, some individuals benefit from the use of a saliva substitute for periods of 2 to 4 hours.
  - Pilocarpine hydrochloride can reduce symptoms.

Esophagitis and Pharyngitis

- These conditions can be so severe that patients may be unable to swallow or take food. Effects are usually transient.
- The following mixture can be taken to provide relief:
  - Mylanta: 450 mL (three 5-oz bottles)
  - Lidocaine hydrochloride 2% viscous solution: 100 mL
  - Diphenhydramine hydrochloride elixir: 60 mL
  - Shake well and refrigerate. Dosage: 1 to 2 tablespoons 15 minutes before meals and at bedtime
- Encourage high-calorie, high-protein, high-carbohydrate liquids and soft, bland foods (e.g., milk shakes, "instant" liquid meals, supplements).

Chest and Lung
Esophagitis and Pharyngitis

- Hoarseness caused by laryngeal mucous membrane congestion sometimes occurs.
- The patient may complain of feeling a lump in the throat.
- Support measures are similar to those discussed previously.

Pneumonitis

- Radiation pneumonitis may be a transient response to moderate radiation doses.
- Bed rest, bronchial dilators, oxygen therapy, and glucocorticosteroids are the usual approaches.
- Late changes are fibrosis in lung tissue and thickening of pleura.

Abdomen and Pelvis
Nausea and Vomiting

- Nausea and vomiting are not common, but occur when treatment is directed to whole abdomen or portions of it, large pelvic fields, hypochondrium, epigastrium, or paraaortic areas.
- Symptoms usually occur 1 to 3 hours after treatment.
- Patients at risk should be premedicated with antiemetics 1 hour before treatment and then delay intake of a full meal until 3 or 4 hours after treatment.
- Small frequent meals and snacks may help.
- Multiple other factors may be involved, such as medications, chemotherapy, or pain.

Diarrhea and Proctitis

- Diarrhea and proctitis occur if areas of the abdomen and pelvis are treated with high doses of radiation.

- Diarrhea is a result of denuding of the small intestine.
  - Effect ranges from increased number of bowel movements to loose, watery stools and intestinal cramping.
  - Occasionally, treatment is interrupted to allow bowel to recover, especially in elderly or debilitated individuals.
  - A low-residue diet and antidiarrheal agents are usually sufficient to control diarrhea.
  - Intravenous fluids for short-term replacement may be needed.
- Proctitis can be accompanied by tenesmus.
  - Proctitis occurs mostly if the area treated includes the rectum, anus, or prostate.
  - A low residue diet is helpful.
  - Sitz baths and antiinflammatory agents in cream or gel form provide relief. Antispasmodics may reduce tenesmus.

Cystitis
- Radiation-induced cystitis can occur early but has a transient effect.
- Cystitis usually occurs within 3 to 5 weeks of therapy.
- With high radiation doses, nephritis may occur.
- Treatment consists of urinary antiseptics and antispasmodics for symptomatic relief.
- High fluid intake is encouraged.
- Sitz baths may be contraindicated if the perineal area is being irradiated.

Reproductive System
The cervix and uterine body are radioresistant. The mucosa of the area is radiosensitive.

Vaginitis
- The vaginal mucous membrane response to radiation is mucositis and inflammation, causing dryness, pruritus, and mucosal discharge.

- Vaginal lubricants are advised until the reaction subsides.
- Vaginal stenosis may be the late result of brachytherapy.

Sterility

- Radiation to the ovaries may produce temporary or permanent sterility, depending on age of person being treated and the radiation dose.
- Hormonal changes and early menopause may occur after radiation of the ovaries. Hormone replacement therapy is controversial.
- Genetic damage may occur after radiation of the gonads in both males and females. Radiation to male testes damages and prevents maturation of sperm.
- Sterility may be permanent even in low doses. Sperm banking and in vitro fertilization are options.

Effects on the embryo and fetus can range from death to abnormalities, including growth or mental retardation, microencephaly, spina bifida, hydrocephalus, blindness, clubfoot, and scalp alopecia.

Total Body Radiation Syndrome

Doses of 150 to 2000 cGy delivered to the whole body in a short time (hours or days) produce life-shortening or lethal damage, particularly to the hematopoietic system, gastrointestinal tract, and cerebrovascular system.

Radiation-Induced Malignancies

Radiation carcinogenesis depends on a number of variables, such as the latent period (usually 1 to 30 years), radiation dose, and radiation-induced tissue or cellular injury. Malignancies that have been associated with radiation are skin cancer, leukemia, sarcoma, thyroid cancer, and lung cancer.

PART III

Chapter 11
....

Chemotherapy

PART I. PRINCIPLES OF CHEMOTHERAPY

Factors Affecting Response to Chemotherapy

Researchers have only recently begun to identify the primary pharmacological activity of many antineoplastic agents. The following factors affect response to chemotherapy.

The Cell Cycle

The cell cycle is made up of five phases, which describe periods of time for different cell processes that result in cell death or reproduction:

- G_1: Synthesis of RNA and proteins (time is variable)
- S: DNA is replicated (10–20 hours)
- G_2: Cell prepares for division (2–10 hours)
- M: Mitosis-cell divides (30–60 minutes)
- G_0: Following mitosis, the cell may either leave the cell cycle and die, enter G_1 phase and cycle again, or rest in the G_0 phase. Cells in the resting phase are resistant to cytotoxic effects of chemotherapy.

Tumor Cell Kinetics

Tumor cells are different from normal cells because they do not stop dividing, they lack differentiation, they can invade local tissues, and they can establish new growths at distant sites. Tumor cells accumulate because their proliferation exceeds cell death.

Biological Characteristics of Tumors
Tumor factors such as growth and size influence response to chemotherapy.

- Actively dividing cells are most sensitive to chemotherapy.
- Tumor cells vary in their sensitivity to chemotherapy.
- Large tumors have small growth fractions and are less responsive.
- Tumor cells can mutate, becoming resistant over time to chemotherapy.

Host Characteristics
Patient factors
- Nutritional status and age
- Level of immune function
- Organ dysfunction
- Physical and psychological tolerance to treatment
- Response to supportive therapies

Drug Factors
Response to a specific drug or drug regimen is related to
- dose and schedule of administration,
- toxicity of drug, and
- route of administration.

Drug Resistance
Cytotoxic drug resistance is a major factor in response to chemotherapy. Drug resistance arises from spontaneous genetic mutations. *Primary* drug resistance is present prior to treatment. *Secondary* drug resistance develops after exposure to chemotherapy.

Therapeutic Strategies

Combination Chemotherapy
The use of multiple agents with different actions may

- provide maximal cell kill for resistant cells,
- minimize development of resistant cells, and
- provide maximum cell kill with tolerable toxicity.

Scheduling and Drug Sequencing

Measures to prevent acquired drug resistance include

- administering intermittent high doses of drugs,
- alternating noncross-resistant chemotherapy regimens,
- minimizing the interval between treatments to coincide with recovery of normal cells, and
- maintaining optimum duration of therapy without dose reductions or treatment delays.

Dose

Dose reductions and treatment delays most often account for suboptimal response to chemotherapy. Critical aspects of dosing include the following factors:

- Dose size refers to the amount of drug delivered to the patient when corrected for physiological variables, such as creatinine clearance and weight.
- Total dose is the sum of all doses of drug for an individual.
- Dose intensity is the amount of drug delivered per unit of time ($mg/m^2/week$).

Reversing Multidrug Resistance

Multidrug resistance occurs when exposure to a single drug is followed by cross-resistance to other drugs. Major strategies to overcome multidrug resistance include the following:

- Increasing intracellular drug concentration using high doses of drugs
- Using chemoprotective agents to permit higher doses of chemotherapy. Examples of such agents include

- amifostine (reduces DNA damage in the kidney in patients receiving cisplatin therapy and may reduce neuropathies as well),
- dexrazoxane (inhibits free radical formation in patients receiving doxorubicin therapy),
- leucovorin (rescues normal cells from toxicity associated with methotrexate), and
- mesna (protects the bladder in patients receiving ifosfamide or cyclophosphamide).
- Combining high doses of chemotherapy with peripheral blood stem cell transplant
- Alternating noncross-resistant chemotherapy regimens
- Using monoclonal antibodies
- Administering chemotherapy according to the patient's circadian rhythm to maximize therapeutic effect and minimize toxicity
- Liposomal encapsulation of doxorubicin and daunorubicin allows a longer half-life and increased uptake by tumor cells, with less toxicity.

New Targets for Anticancer Therapy

New agents are being developed to target tumor cells by other mechanisms that are not toxic to normal cells. These include

- angiogenesis inhibitors that limit tumor growth and include angiostatin, endostatin, thalidomide, and antivascular endothelial growth factor; and
- matrix metalloproteinase inhibitors, which prevent enzymes from promoting tumor cell metastasis.

Cancer Chemotherapy Drug Development

Clinical Trials

Following initial development, new drugs must be tested in humans via clinical trials to evaluate

PART III

their activity and toxicity. A clinical trial is a scientific study conducted according to a written guideline for the study (protocol). See Chapter 8 for a discussion of the different phases of clinical trials.

Pharmacology of Chemotherapeutic Drugs

Principles of Pharmacokinetics

Pharmacokinetics is the study of the movement of drugs in the body. There are four major principles to consider:

1. **Absorption:** The amount of drug that reaches the circulation and the tumor depends on the degree to which the drug is absorbed.
2. **Distribution:** Distribution is determined primarily by the drug's ability to penetrate different tissues and bind to various plasma proteins.
3. **Metabolism:** Metabolic activation and inactivation or catabolism of drugs is carried out primarily by the liver.
4. **Elimination:** The kidneys are responsible for the majority of the elimination of drugs and drug metabolites.

Antineoplastic Drugs

Cancer chemotherapeutic drugs have traditionally been classified by their mechanisms of action, chemical structure, or biologic source.

Alkylating Agents

These agents are cell cycle nonspecific and are most active in the resting phase (G_0). Examples include

- nitrogen mustard,
- carboplatin,
- cyclophosphamide,
- ifosfamide,

- melphalan,
- dacarbazine, and
- lomustine.

Antitumor Antibiotics
These agents are cell cycle nonspecific. Examples include

- bleomycin,
- doxorubicin,
- mitomycin C,
- mitoxantrone, and
- daunorubicin.

Antimetabolites
These agents are cell cycle specific and interfere with DNA synthesis. Examples include

- methotrexate,
- mercaptopurine,
- 5-fluorouracil,
- cytarabine,
- gemcitabine,
- trimetrexate, and
- cladribine.

Plant Derivatives
Many of the drugs in this group were isolated from plant material. Others are analogues of compounds extracted from plants. These drugs interfere with mitotic activity and are cell cycle specific.

- Vinca alkaloids
  - vincristine
  - teniposide
  - vinblastine
  - vindesine
  - etoposide
  - vinorelbine

- Taxanes
  - paclitaxel
  - docetaxel
- Camptothecin analogues
  - topotecan
  - irinotecan

Hormonal Therapy

These agents probably inhibit specific receptors. Blocking these receptors prevents the cell from receiving hormonal growth stimulation. Examples include the following:

- Antiestrogens: tamoxifen, toremifen
- Aromatase inhibitors: anastrozole, letrozole
- Gonadotropin-releasing hormone analogues: leuprolide, goserelin
- Antiandrogens: flutamide, nilutamide, bicalutamide

Appendixes A and B provide detailed information on oral and intravenous antineoplastic agents.

PART II. CHEMOTHERAPY: PRINCIPLES OF ADMINISTRATION

Chemotherapy Administration

Professional Qualifications

Basic qualifications for nurses administering antineoplastic agents include the following:

- Current licensure as registered nurse
- Certification in CPR
- Intravenous therapy skills
- Educational preparation and demonstration of knowledge in all areas related to antineoplastic drugs
- Drug administration skills
- Policies and procedures to govern nursing actions:

- Chemotherapy drug preparation and handling guidelines that comply with Occupational Safety and Health Administration guidelines
- Chemotherapy administration procedures
- Vesicant management
- Management of allergic reactions
- Safe drug handling and disposal
- Patient and family education
- Management of vascular access devices (VADs)
- Documentation methods
- Outcome standards
- Oncology quality improvement process

PART III

Handling Cytotoxic Drugs

Exposure to cytotoxic drugs is potentially hazardous. All chemotherapy drugs should be prepared under a class II biological safety hood. Personal protective equipment (PPE) is worn during handling of chemotherapeutic agents. All sharps, containers, and cytotoxic waste must be disposed according to state and federal guidelines. Any spills or direct exposure should be documented and monitored.

Patient and Family Education

Nurses are responsible for giving the patient and family specific information about cancer and its treatment. Some basic teaching principles include the following:

- Identify specific learning needs related to chemotherapy.
- Prepare teaching aids such as written materials, calendars, video, and teaching guides.
- Describe various sensations that the patient will experience during treatment (e.g., stuffy nose, lightheadedness, dizziness).
- Describe specific side effects and measures to prevent complications.

- Teach patients self-care measures and give clear instructions on how to report symptoms.
- Ensure that informed consent has been obtained.
- Document the teaching in the patient's medical record and describe the method of follow-up.

Administration Principles
Dose Calculation
- Dose of drug is based on body surface area (mg/m^2) or milligrams per kilogram.
- Obese patients may require a dose adjustment. Dose may be based on the average of their actual weight and their ideal weight.
- The Calvert formula is based on physiologic function and seeks to deliver the optimal dose of carboplatin based on the creatinine clearance, age, history of prior chemotherapy, and goal of therapy.

Steps to Administer an Antineoplastic Drug
- Verify the patient's identity.
- Check and double-check the drug order.
- Calculate body surface area to confirm dosage.
- Ensure that informed consent has been obtained.
- Evaluate laboratory results.
- Locate the extravasation kit or supplies, if giving vesicant.
- Wash hands, don gloves, and other PPE.
- Select the equipment and site for venipuncture.
- Use an appropriate sterile technique for venous access.
- Tape the needle securely, without obstructing the site.
- Test the vein with at least 5 to 8 cc of normal saline.
- Administer chemotherapy with an even, steady pressure.

- Check for blood return every couple of cubic centimeters (milliliters) of drug given.
- Flush between each drug to avoid incompatibilities.
- When the injection or infusion is complete, dispose of all equipment according to the policies and procedures of the institution.
- Arrange for follow-up care.
- Document the procedure in the patient's medical record.

Preventing Drug Errors

- Verbal orders are never given or taken for chemotherapy drugs.
- The physician responsible for the care of the patient and most familiar with the drug and dosing schedule should write the chemotherapy orders.
- Avoid abbreviations, especially for similar sounding and spelled drugs (e.g., mitomycin and mitoxantrone, vinorelbine and vinblastine, 5-FU and 5-FUdr).
- The drug name, dose in mg/m^2 (if appropriate), total daily dose, and cumulative dose should be written.
- Only the drug order as written by the physician should be used by the pharmacist to prepare the label for the drug.
- All orders are checked by the pharmacist against previous orders.
- Variations from previous drug orders are verified.
- Avoid the use of extraneous zeros, as this leads to errors in which 100.0 becomes 1000. It is better to spell out the amount rather than depend on interpretation.
- Drugs are dispensed in large trays or large z-lock bags to contain the drug and avoid confusing one patient's drugs with another's.
- The individual giving the drug should not be the same person who prepared the drug unless

another individual has double checked the order.

- All persons handling chemotherapy should be properly trained.
- Policies and procedures for drug preparation and administration should be updated once a year.

Vesicant Extravasation

Vesicant drugs can cause tissue necrosis if they infiltrate soft tissue from a blood vessel. Irritant drugs cause localized irritation, even burning, but no tissue necrosis if infiltrated. Table 11.1 lists vesicant drugs and drugs that are irritating to the vein on administration.

Extravasation of a vesicant can result in physical deformity or functional deficit. Measures to minimize risk of extravasation include the following:

- Identify patients at risk: the patients who are unable to communicate clearly, the elderly, and confused, debilitated patients with frail, fragile veins.
- Avoid infusing vesicants over joints, bony prominences, tendons, or antecubital fossa.

Table 11.1 Vesicant and Irritant Drugs	
Vesicants	**Irritants**
Dactinomycin	Carmustine
Daunorubicin	Dacarbazine
Doxorubicin	Docetaxel
Estramustine	Etoposide
Idarubicin	Doxorubicin liposomal
Mitomycin C	Mithramycin
Nitrogen mustard	Mitoxantrone
Teniposide	Paclitaxel
Vinblastine	Streptozocin
Vincristine	Vinorelbine

- Avoid giving vesicant drugs in areas where venous or lymphatic circulation is poor.
- Give the vesicant agent before other agents.
- If a vesicant is ordered as an infusion, it is given only through a central line.
- Have available an extravasation kit and all materials necessary to manage extravasation.

Symptoms of extravasation include

- swelling at the injection site;
- stinging, burning, or pain at the injection site;
- redness; and
- lack of blood return.

If extravasation is suspected, stop the infusion and follow official policy and procedure for extravasation.

Routes of Drug Administration
- Topical
- Oral
- Intramuscular
- Subcutaneous
- Intravenous
- Intrathecal
- Intraperitoneal
- Intrapleural
- Intravesical

Vascular Access Devices
There are many different types of catheters, needles, and implantable ports for the delivery of cancer chemotherapy. The nurse will assess and help select or recommend the proper device. Some of the major vascular access device types and features are summarized.

Nontunneled Central Venous Catheters
- Indicated for short-term use
- Multilumen catheter permits polydrug therapy

- Easily removed
- Sterile technique used during care

Tunneled Central Venous Catheters
- Indicated for frequent intravenous access
- Cuff surrounds catheter, permitting fibrous ingrowth
- Requires sterile site care with dressings until formation of granulation tissue (about 7 days)
- Requires flushing every other day or weekly (Groshong catheter)
- Flush with 3 to 5 cc of heparinized saline (10 to 100 U/mL).
- Avoid intraluminal mixing of potentially incompatible drugs by flushing with saline between each drug.

Implantable Ports
- Completely implanted under skin
- Permits access to venous or arterial system or peritoneal, pleural, or epidural space
- Accessed by noncoring needle

Complication Management
Intraluminal Catheter Occlusion
Complication arises from

- blood clot within catheter,
- crystallization or precipitate, and
- improper needle placement in the port (low-profile ports require a three-fourths-inch 22-gauge needle, not a 1-inch needle).

Prevention and management

- Maintain positive pressure during the flush.
- Avoid excessive manipulation of the catheter.
- Vigorously flush with 20 cc (mL) saline after the blood draw.
- Flush between each drug to prevent incompatibility.

- Flush every 8 to 12 hours when giving total parenteral nutrition (TPN) or lipids.
- If a blood clot is suspected, instill alteplase (tPA) 2 mg/mL. Allow it to dwell for 2 hours; then attempt to aspirate.

Extraluminal Catheter Occlusion

Complication arises from

- fibrin sheath formation,
- thrombosis,
- catheter position, and
- pinch-off syndrome.

Prevention and management

- Vigorously flush to prevent fibrin sheath formation.
- Lyse the fibrin sheath with urokinase with a dwell time of 24 hours.
- Low-dose warfarin may prevent or decrease incidence of thrombus formation.
- Anticoagulants may be necessary to treat venous thrombosis.

Infection

Manifestations

- Infection is most common in patients with neutropenia and/or multilumen catheters and in those receiving TPN.
- Local skin infections are common.
- Symptoms include redness, warmth, discomfort, exudates, and fever.

Prevention and management

- Provide meticulous catheter care.
- Obtain a culture of the area.
- Increase the frequency of catheter care.
- Administer appropriate antibiotics.
- Take blood cultures (intraluminal and peripheral).

PART III

PART III. MANAGEMENT OF CHEMOTHERAPY TOXICITIES

Virtually every organ is affected by chemotherapy. Interventions focus on preventing or minimizing toxicities.

Pretreatment Evaluation

It is important to assess risk factors before initiating therapy. Vigorous treatment is not tolerated in the following cases:

- Patients in weak physical condition
- Patients with poor nutritional status
- Heavily pretreated patients who may lack marrow reserve, placing them at higher risk for infection, bleeding, or anemia
- Individuals who are unable or unwilling to care for themselves
- Patients with preexisting hepatic or renal dysfunction, which can alter absorption, distribution, metabolism, and elimination of drugs
- Patients with hypovolemia and dehydration from nausea, vomiting, or diarrhea, which may increase the risk of acute renal failure
- Patients with a concomitant illness that affects their ability to metabolize the drug or to care for themselves
- Patients for whom compliance with the treatment program may be influenced by financial and third-party payment concerns

Patient Education and Follow-Up

The goals of chemotherapy teaching include

- helping the patient adjust to treatment,
- explaining how the treatment will affect the cancer,
- imparting the sequence of administration,
- recognizing and controlling side effects,
- encouraging self-care behaviors that minimize side effects, and

- listing side effects to report to the health care professional.

Grading of Toxicities

Grading is a means of standardization of assessment and documentation of side effects. To assess toxicity, knowledge of the following is necessary:

- Which toxicities occurred
- Toxicity severity
- Time of onset
- Duration of effect
- Interventions used to minimize effect

Systemic Toxicities

Bone Marrow Suppression

Myelosuppression is the most common dose-limiting side effect of chemotherapy. The point of lowest blood count (nadir) occurs about 7 to 14 days after chemotherapy. Alkylating agents and nitrosoureas are most toxic, while antimetabolites, vinca alkaloids, and antitumor antibiotics are less toxic.

Risk factors

- Tumor cells in bone marrow
- Prior treatment with chemotherapy or radiation
- Poor nutrition

Maturation of cells in the bone marrow takes 8 to 10 days, with variation in the life span for each cell type.

Thrombocytopenia

- The life span of platelets is 7 to 10 days.
- Thrombocytopenia occurs on days 8 to 14.
- Manifestations of thrombocytopenia include
  - easy bruising,
  - bleeding from gums, nose, or other orifices, and

  - petechiae on extremities and pressure points.
- Platelet transfusions are indicated if the platelet count drops quickly to a dangerous level (20,000/mm³ or less) or if the patient is bleeding.

Anemia
- Red blood cells have a life span of 120 days.
- Manifestations of anemia include
  - pallor,
  - fatigue,
  - hypotension,
  - tachycardia,
  - headache,
  - tachypnea, and
  - irritability.
- Transfusions are indicated when
  - hemoglobin goes below 8 g/100 mL,
  - the patient is symptomatic (e.g., short of breath), and
  - the patient is bleeding.
- Consideration should be given to the growth factor erythropoietin.

Neutropenia
- The life span of granulocytes is 6 to 8 hours.
- Neutropenia usually develops 8 to 12 days after chemotherapy.
- Chemotherapy is often withheld if the white blood cell (WBC) count is below 3000/mm³ or if the absolute neutrophil count (ANC) is below 1500/mm³.
- Profound neutropenia (grade 4) is defined as an ANC of less than 500 cells/mm³.
- ANC is calculated by multiplying the WBC count by the neutrophil count (segmented neutrophils + bands) × WBC = ANC.

- Infections from invasion and overgrowth of pathogenic microbes increase in frequency and severity as ANC decreases.
- Risk of severe infections increases when the nadir persists for more than 7 to 10 days.
- Chemotherapy-induced damage to alimentary canal and respiratory tract mucosa facilitates entry of infecting organisms; 80% of infections arise from endogenous microbial flora.
- When the neutrophil count is less than 500 cells/mm^3, approximately 20% or more of febrile episodes are accompanied by bacteremia caused principally by aerobic gram-negative bacilli and gram-positive cocci.
- Treatment involves culture and broad-spectrum antibiotics for a minimum of 7 days.
- Fever persisting for more than 3 days without identification of the infected site or organism suggests
  - a nonbacterial cause (may begin antifungal therapy),
  - resistance to the antibiotic,
  - emergence of a second bacterial infection,
  - inadequate antibiotic serum and tissue levels,
  - drug fever, or
  - infection at an avascular site (abscess).
- Colony-stimulating factors can shorten the duration of neutropenia.

Fatigue

Fatigue is the most common and distressing side effect of chemotherapy. The cause of fatigue in a cancer patient is unknown but may relate to

- changes in musculoskeletal protein stores,
- metabolite concentration and accumulation,
- changes in energy usage or disease pattern,
- anemia and psychological distress, and

- metabolism of end products of cellular destruction by chemotherapy.

Manifestations of fatigue include weariness, weakness, and lack of energy. See Chapter 18 for interventions to overcome fatigue.

Gastrointestinal Toxicities

Diarrhea

Diarrhea results from destruction of actively dividing epithelial cells of the gastrointestinal (GI) tract. Degree and duration of diarrhea depend on

- drugs (e.g., 5-FU, methotrexate),
- dose,
- nadir, and
- frequency of chemotherapy.

Without adequate management, prolonged diarrhea will cause

- dehydration,
- nutritional malabsorption, and
- circulatory collapse.

Management often includes the following:

- Temporary discontinuation of chemotherapy
- A low-residue, high-calorie, high-protein diet
- Pharmacological measures
  - Anticholinergic drugs to reduce gastric secretions and decrease intestinal peristalsis
  - Opiate therapy to slow down intestinal motility and increase fluid absorption
  - Octreotide acetate, which prolongs intestinal transit time, increasing intestinal water and electrolyte transport and decreasing GI blood-flow
- Stool cultures to rule out infectious process
- Antidiarrheal agents are not given to counteract diarrhea resulting from infection, because these agents promote slow passage of stool through the intestines, prolonging mucosal exposure to the organism's toxins.

Constipation

Infrequent, excessively hard and dry bowel movements result from a decrease in rectal filling or emptying. Risk factors include

- narcotic analgesics,
- a decrease in physical activity,
- a low-fiber diet,
- a decrease in fluid intake,
- poor dentition in the elderly population,
- bed rest, and
- diminished rectal emptying caused by vincristine or vinblastine therapy; these drugs cause autonomic nerve dysfunction.

Prevention of constipation includes the following:

- A prophylactic stool softener before beginning vincristine or vinblastine therapy
- An increase in fiber, fluids, and physical activity
- Notify the physician if more than 3 days have passed without a bowel movement, because impaction, ileus, or obstipation can occur.

Nausea and Vomiting

The management of chemotherapy-related nausea and vomiting has vastly improved. Emesis can be induced by

- stimulation of the vomiting center (VC);
- obstruction, irritation, inflammation, or delayed gastric emptying; and
- conditioned anticipatory responses.

Although nausea, retching, and vomiting commonly occur together, they are separate conditions.

- Nausea
  - Subjective, conscious recognition of the urge to vomit
  - Manifested by unpleasant, wavelike sensation in the epigastric area, at back of throat, or throughout the abdomen

- Mediated by autonomic nervous system and accompanied by symptoms such as tachycardia, perspiration, lightheadedness, dizziness, pallor, excess salivation, and weakness
- Retching
  - Rhythmic and spasmodic movement involving the diaphragm and abdominal muscles
  - Controlled by the respiratory center in the brainstem near the VC
  - Negative intrathoracic pressure and positive abdominal pressure result in unproductive retching.
  - When negative pressure becomes positive, vomiting occurs.
- Vomiting
  - Somatic process performed by respiratory muscles causing forceful oral expulsion of gastric, duodenal, or jejunal contents.

Classifications of nausea and vomiting

- *Acute:* nausea and vomiting 1 to 2 hours after treatment
- *Delayed:* nausea and vomiting persisting or developing 24 hours after chemotherapy; less common if acute emesis is prevented
- *Anticipatory:* nausea and vomiting occurring as a result of classic operant conditioning from stimuli associated with chemotherapy
- *Conditioned responses* experienced after a few sessions of chemotherapy; occurs most commonly when efforts to control emesis are unsuccessful

Risk factors

- Emetic potential of drug(s)
- Onset and duration of emetic response
- Dose of drug
- Schedule of drug
- Age: younger patients more susceptible

- Prior chemotherapy
- Anxiety
- Gender: women more than men

Management strategies

- Treat prophylactically before chemotherapeutic treatment.
- Use a combination antiemetic therapy (e.g., serotonin antagonist such as granisetron, ondansetron, or dolasetron, plus dexamethasone or solu medrol and compazine with or without a sedative for sleep).
- Employ behavior strategies (e.g., progressive muscle relaxation, hypnosis, and systematic desensitization).

Mucous Membranes

Mucositis is a general term that describes the inflammatory response of mucosal epithelial cells to cytotoxic effects of chemotherapy (i.e., oral cavity [stomatitis], esophagus [esophagitis], intestines [enteritis], vagina [vaginitis]).

Risk factors

- Hematological malignancies
- Age: younger patients more than older patients
- Preexisting oral disease
- Poor oral hygiene
- Local irritants: tobacco, alcohol
- Chemotherapeutic agents: bleomycin, doxorubicin, daunorubicin, 5-FU, methotrexate, taxanes, and high-dose chemotherapy
- Radiation to the oral cavity
- Infections (e.g., bacterial, fungal, and viral)

Prevention

- Frequent oral hygiene, including flossing
- Hydration
- Gum massage
- Ice chips during chemotherapy administration

Mucositis and stomatitis are commonly associated with

- painful ulceration,
- hemorrhage, and
- secondary infection.

Treatment is symptom related:

- A stomatitis cocktail with mylanta, viscous xylocaine, and benadryl is soothing as a swish and swallow.
- Tylenol with or without codeine or other pain medication is appropriate for more intense pain.

Taste Alterations

Alterations in food perception, taste, and smell are commonly caused by chemotherapy. The following chemotherapy drugs are associated with taste alteration:

- Cyclophosphamide
- Dacarbazine
- Doxorubicin
- 5-FU
- Levamisole
- Methotrexate
- Nitrogen mustard
- Cisplatin
- Vincristine

Nursing interventions are aimed at self-care to maintain optimal nutrition.

Integument

Hyperpigmentation

Discoloration of skin, nails, and mucous membranes are associated with 5-FU, busulfan, cyclophosphamide, and bleomycin.

Hypersensitivity

Cutaneous hypersensitivity reactions (HSRs) to chemotherapy occur infrequently. Immediate

HSRs generally present as urticaria, angioedema, or anaphylaxis. Hypersensitivity can occur with many drugs, namely paclitaxel, docetaxel, cisplatin, carboplatin, and teniposide.

Acral Erythema

Painful erythema, scaling, and epidermal sloughing from the palms and soles are associated with continuous infusions of 5-FU, doxorubicin, paclitaxel and high-dose cytarabine, and floxuridine.

Photosensitivity

An enhanced skin response to ultraviolet rays occurs most commonly with 5-FU, dacarbazine, vinblastine, and high-dose methotrexate.

Alopecia

Alopecia is the most noticeable and often most distressing side effect. Hair loss depends on the dose of the drug, amount of drug used, and route of administration. Patients are given a prescription for a "cranial prosthesis" for chemotherapy alopecia for insurance reimbursement.

Organ Toxicity

Cardiotoxicity

Acute cardiac toxicity

- Characterized by transient changes on electrocardiogram (ECG)
- Occurs in about 10% of patients receiving chemotherapy

Chronic cardiac toxicity

- Characterized by onset of symptoms weeks or months after therapy
- Cardiomyopathy is irreversible.
- Congestive heart failure presents as a low-voltage QRS complex.
- Fewer than 5% of patients develop chronic cardiotoxicity.

Signs and symptoms

- Nonproductive cough
- Dyspnea
- Pedal edema
- Tachycardia

Risk factors

- Anthracyclines directly damage the myocyte of the heart.
- Total cumulative doses of 550 mg/m^2 of doxorubicin, 600 mg/m^2 of daunomycin, and 400 mg/m^2 of epirubicin
- If mediastinal radiation has been given, the dose of doxorubicin is reduced to 450 mg/m^2.
- High doses of cyclophosphamide or 5-FU increase the risk for cardiac damage.
- Cardiotoxicity is increased in patients receiving Herceptin if they have had prior doxorubicin and cyclophosphamide.

Prevention

- Limit the total dose of anthracycline.
- Low-dose continuous infusions minimize cardiac toxicity.
- Administer chemoprotectants if appropriate.
- Use fewer cardiotoxic analogues if possible.

Management

- Monitor the ECG and radionuclide scan to evaluate heart function.
- Instruct the patient to conserve energy.
- Manage fluid retention and minimize sodium intake.
- Digitalis therapy may enhance cardiac output.
- Diuretics may be useful to decrease cardiac load.
- Oxygen may be useful to manage dyspnea.

Neurotoxicity

Chemotherapy-induced neurotoxicity may result in direct or indirect damage to the central nervous system (CNS), peripheral nervous system, cranial nerves, or any combination of these.

- CNS damage produces altered reflexes, unsteady gait, ataxia, and confusion.
- Peripheral nervous system damage produces paralysis or loss of movement and sensation to those areas affected by the particular nerve.
- Autonomic nervous system damage causes ileus, impotence, or urinary retention.

Drugs most commonly associated with neurotoxicity and their associated symptoms

- Vincristine
  - Peripheral neuropathy
  - Myalgias, loss of deep tendon reflexes at the ankle, progressing to complete areflexia
  - Distal symmetric sensory loss, motor weakness, footdrop, and muscle atrophy
  - Ileus, constipation, impotence, urinary retention, or postural hypotension
- Cisplatin
  - Paresthesias of hands and feet (common)
  - Sensory ataxia
  - High-tone hearing loss
- Paclitaxel
  - Peripheral neuropathy
  - Myalgias and arthralgias (dose-dependent)
  - Autonomic neuropathy
  - Symptoms gradually improve after cessation of therapy.

Other drugs associated with neurotoxicity

- Ifosfamide
- High-dose methotrexate
- High-dose cytarabine

- 5-FU
- Vinorelbine

Prevention and management strategies

- Neurological assessment before treatment
- Dose modification may be necessary to prevent irreversible damage.
- Celebrex, vicoprofen, and Vioxx may be used to minimize pain associated with myalgias with taxanes.
- Vinorelbine causes pain and aching in the treatment arm when given as a peripheral infusion. The patient requires a central line access to continue vinorelbine.

Pulmonary Toxicity

Chemotherapy can damage endothelial cells, resulting in pneumonitis. Long-term exposure to chemotherapy causes extensive alteration of pulmonary parenchyma.

Risk factors

- Age: very young and elderly
- Preexisting lung disease
- History of smoking
- Cumulative dose
- Long-term therapy
- Mediastinal radiation
- High inspired concentration of oxygen

Drugs commonly associated with pulmonary toxicity

- Bleomycin: cumulative dose should not exceed 400 to 450 U; it induces interstitial changes with hyperplasia.
- Cytarabine directly damages pneumocytes.
- Mitomycin C causes diffuse alveolar damage.
- Cyclophosphamide causes endothelial swelling.

Presenting symptoms

- Dyspnea
- Bilateral basilar rales

- Unproductive cough
- Tachypnea
- Low-grade fever
- Tachycardia
- Wheezing
- Pleural rub
- Fatigue

Management
- Conservation of energy
- Corticosteroids
- Diuretics

Hepatotoxicity

Chemotherapy can cause a variety of hepatotoxic reactions. Obstruction to hepatic blood flow results in fatty changes, hepatocellular necrosis, and veno-occlusive disease.

Risk factors
- Increased age
- Prior liver damage (e.g., hepatitis)
- Elevated serum glutamic oxaloacetic transaminase (SGOT) level
- Alcoholism

Chemotherapy drugs commonly associated with liver toxicity

- Methotrexate
- Nitrosoureas
- 6-Mercaptopurine
- Etoposide (high dose)
- Cisplatin (high dose)
- Cytarabine
- Cyclophosphamide (high dose)
- Paclitaxel
- Docetaxel
- Gemcitabine

Symptoms
- Elevated liver function test results
- Chemical hepatitis
- Jaundice
- Abdominal pain
- Hepatomegaly
- Ascites
- Decreased albumin level
- Cirrhosis

Management
- Monitor liver function tests.
- Reduce doses in the presence of liver dysfunction for drugs metabolized in the liver.
- Avoid alcohol intake.

Hemorrhagic Cystitis
A bladder toxicity resulting from damage to the bladder mucosa caused by acrolein, a metabolite of cyclophosphamide and ifosfamide
Symptoms
- Microscopic hematuria
- Transient irritative urination
- Dysuria
- Suprapubic pain
- Hemorrhage

Risk factors
- High doses of ifosfamide or cyclophosphamide

Prevention and management
- Adequate hydration
- Frequent bladder emptying
- Mesna therapy
- Testing of urine for occult blood (Hemastik)

Nephrotoxicity
Damage to kidneys is caused by either direct renal cell damage or obstructive nephropathy

(i.e., tumor lysis syndrome or uric acid nephropathy).

Risk factors

- Elderly patient
- Preexisting renal disease
- Poor nutritional status
- Dehydration
- Large tumor mass
- High cumulative dose of nephrotoxic drug
- Concomitant administration of aminoglycoside therapy

Symptoms

- Increased blood urea nitrogen and creatinine
- Oliguria
- Azotemia
- Proteinuria
- Hyperuricemia
- Hypomagnesemia
- Hypocalcemia

Drugs commonly associated with nephrotoxicity

- Cisplatin: Damages renal cells
- Methotrexate: Damage occurs because drug precipitates out in an acid environment to obstruct renal tubules.
- Streptozocin: Directly damages tubules, causing tubular atrophy
- Nitrosoureas: Causes delayed renal failure (azotemia and proteinuria followed by progressive renal failure)
- Mitomycin C: Renal failure and microangiopathic hemolytic anemia occur in approximately 20% of patients who have received a cumulative dose of 100 mg or more.

Prevention

- Evaluate the patient's renal status before therapy.
- Adequately hydrate the patient.

- Encourage the patient to drink 3 L of fluid per day.
- Decrease uric acid production with allopurinol in patients with high tumor load.
- Ensure that the patient receiving methotrexate has pretreatment with sodium bicarbonate to alkalinize the urine.
- Use of mannitol induces diuresis with cisplatin therapy.
- Use of amifostine to reduce the cumulative renal toxicity associated with repeated cisplatin therapy.

Gonadal Toxicity

Chemotherapy effects on the gonads include gonadal failure, infertility, and premature menopause.

Risk factors

- Age: Women over 30 are less likely to regain ovarian function because they have fewer oocytes than do younger women.
- Cycle nonspecific agents are most toxic and include
  - busulfan,
  - melphalan,
  - nitrogen mustard,
  - procarbazine, and
  - chlorambucil.
- Drug-induced testicular damage results in azospermia, oligospermia, and abnormalities of semen volume and motility. Sperm banking is an option for men to preserve their ability to produce children.

Secondary and Therapy-Related Cancers

Long-term survivors are at highest risk for a second primary cancer. Alkylating agents are most often implicated as risk factors for second malignancies. Long-term survivors and their children should be monitored for their lifetimes.

Chapter 12
. . . .

Principles of Bone Marrow and Hematopoietic Cell Transplantation

---

PART I. PRINCIPLES OF TRANSPLANTATION

Types of Transplantation

Different types of hematopoietic cell transplantation are described in terms of the hematopoietic stem cell source.

- *Syngeneic:* Donor is an identical twin (perfect human leukocyte antigen (HLA) match.
- *Allogeneic:* Depends on the availability of an HLA-matched donor. The closer the HLA match between donor and recipient, the better. A related donor is preferred.
- *Autologous:* Stem cell donor is the patient.
- *Umbilical cord:* Used as stem cell source for both related and unrelated donor transplants

Transplantation Indications

Leukemias continue to be the most frequent diagnosis treated with the allogeneic transplant. High-dose chemotherapy and autologous stem cell rescue have been used to treat solid tumors. Malignant diseases treated with transplantation include the following:

- *Hematological malignancies:* acute lymphocytic and myelogenous leukemia, chronic lymphocytic and myelogenous leukemia, myelodysplastic syndrome, non-Hodgkin's lymphoma, Hodgkin's disease, multiple myeloma

- *Solid tumors:* breast cancer, neuroblastoma, testicular germ cell tumors, lung cancer, brain tumor, ovarian cancer, melanoma, sarcoma

A variety of congenital and acquired nonmalignant diseases are treated with allogeneic transplantation.

Standards for Transplantation

The Foundation for the Accreditation of Hematopoietic Cell Therapy (FAHCT) was established in 1996 and standards were published. A program seeking accreditation must perform at least 10 transplants of each type during the year prior to which accreditation is requested. Nurses must be formally trained and experienced in the management of transplant patients.

The National Marrow Donor Program is a registry of volunteers willing to donate marrow.

The International Bone Marrow Transplant Registry maintains a data base of procedures performed and their outcomes.

Contemporary Issues

Financial and reimbursement controversies exist. Costs of a transplant procedure range from $50,000 to $100,000 or more, depending on the type, complexity, and institutional charging structure.

Various models of care have developed that provide patients with early discharge and care in the outpatient or home setting.

PART II. TECHNIQUES OF HEMATOPOIETIC CELL TRANSPLANTATION

To determine whether the patient is a candidate for transplantation and which type of transplant, a physical, psychosocial, and financial evaluation is done. Extensive education is provided throughout the process.

Cells for Transplantation

The process of obtaining stem cells for transplantation differs according to the type of transplant. With bone marrow transplant (BMT), the cells are obtained through bone marrow harvest. In a blood cell transplant (BCT), the stem cells and progenitor cells are collected from the peripheral blood. Each procedure has its unique steps.

Bone Marrow Harvest

- *Allogeneic:* Replacement marrow is obtained from a related or unrelated HLA-matched donor. The bone marrow harvest is done under anesthesia and obtained from the iliac crests. The cells are given to the patient as soon as possible.
- *Autologous:* The process for obtaining bone marrow is the same as for the allogeneic harvest. The volume may be greater if there is a need to remove tumor cells. The cells are then processed and frozen until needed.

Blood Cell Transplant

This process involves the use of stem cells from the peripheral blood. With BCT, mobilization takes place to release an increased number of peripheral stem cells and progenitor cells. Chemotherapy, hematopoietic growth factors, or both, are used to increase these cells. After mobilization, blood cell separators collect the cells by apheresis.

Cell Processing and Storage

Cells from autologous BMT and BCT are cryopreserved in the same way. Purging of cells may be done to decrease the risk of tumor contamination. Purging is done after the harvest or apheresis and before cryopreservation.

Conditioning Therapy

Conditioning therapy is given to patients to remove any remaining malignant cells. Chemotherapy, total body irradiation, or both, may be used to deplete the marrow. Protocols vary in length from 4 to 7 days before transplant or blood cell reinfusion.

Reinfusion

Reinfusion of bone marrow or peripheral stem cells should occur 24 hours after high-dose chemotherapy. The cells are fragile and should not be manipulated prior to infusion. They are infused immediately, within 10 to 20 minutes of thawing per bag.

PART III. COMPLICATIONS OF TRANSPLANTATION

Both acute and chronic complications can occur in all types of transplants. There are specific complications, however, that occur only in allogeneic transplantation. Complications are generally the result of

- conditioning therapy,
- graft-versus-host disease (GVHD) in allogeneic transplantation,
- problems associated with original disease, and
- adverse effects of medication.

Acute Complications

Acute complications usually occur during the first 100 days. The major acute complications are summarized in the following sections:

Acute Graft-Versus-Host Disease

GVHD is a major complication of allogeneic BMT, occurring in 25% to 80% of patients. The primary organs affected by GVHD are the skin, gastrointestinal tract, and liver.

- Clinical manifestations
  - Maculopapular rash progressing to erythroderma with desquamation

- Profuse diarrhea, nausea, vomiting, abdominal cramping, and gastrointestinal bleeding
- Elevated liver enzymes, hepatosplenomegaly, jaundice
- Prophylaxis and treatment measures
  - Single-agent or combination immunosuppressive agents (e.g., cyclosporine, methotrexate, procarbazine, steroids) reduce the incidence and severity of GVHD.
  - Antibody prophylaxis (e.g., antihuman thymocyte globulin, IL-2) prevents or reduces the severity of GVHD.
  - Cytotoxic agents and glucocorticoids are used to treat diagnostically confirmed GVHD.
  - Gut rest, hyperalimentation, pain control, and antibiotic prophylaxis are routine elements of supportive care for patients with GVHD.

PART III

Infection
Most common infections during the first 3 months posttransplant
- Bacterial
- Fungal (candida, aspergillus)
- Herpes simplex virus
- *Pneumocystis carinii*
- Cytomegalovirus (CMV) infections

Common sites of infection
- Oral cavity
- Gastrointestinal mucosa
- Skin
- Catheter sites

When a patient develops neutropenic fever, empiric antibiotics are started. Acyclovir to prevent herpes simplex virus and ganciclovir to suppress CMV may be given prophylactically.

Gastrointestinal Complications
The majority of patients will experience gastrointestinal toxicity. Nausea, vomiting, anorexia, diar-

rhea, and mucositis are the most common problems.

Venoocclusive Disease

Venoocclusive disease (VOD) is almost exclusive to BMT and occurs during the first few weeks after transplant. It varies from mild disease to severe multiorgan failure. There is no definitive method to prevent VOD.

Clinical manifestations

- Jaundice
- Fluid retention and edema
- Hepatomegaly with liver tenderness
- Increased bilirubin
- Ascites

There is no known specific treatment. Provide supportive care and management of symptoms.

Hematological Complications

Neutropenia may last for 2 to 3 weeks following transplant. Patients receiving BCT may have a shorter period of neutropenia.

Anemia and thrombocytopenia are expected events. Transfusions of irradiated blood products and HLA-matched platelets are required.

Primary graft rejection or failure is the absence of any sign of hematologic function.

Pulmonary Complications

Pneumothorax, pulmonary edema, pulmonary hemorrhage, and pulmonary infections are a major cause of morbidity and mortality, affecting up to 60% of patients.

Cardiac Complications

Cardiac dysfunction can occur in those patients who have received high-dose cyclophosphamide. The clinical picture consists of hemorrhagic cardiomyopathy, congestive heart failure, pericardial effusion, loss of electrocardiogram voltage, and cardiomegaly. Treatment involves symptomatic pharmacologic support and fluid management.

Oral Complications

Almost all patients undergoing blood or marrow transplant develop oral complications. Prophylactic agents and early intervention result in prompt treatment and prolonged survival.

Renal Complications

Renal failure is related to chemotherapy, antibiotics, and cyclosporine given before transplant. Monitoring fluid balance, laboratory values, blood pressure, and medications is essential.

Late Complications

Chronic complications tend to occur 100 days after transplant. Some are transplant-related and others are due to the conditioning regimens or disease recurrence.

Chronic Graft-Versus-Host Disease

Chronic GVHD is the most common late complication in allogeneic transplant recipients. GVHD can develop 2 months to 2 years after transplant. Chronic GVHD affects the skin, liver, eyes, oral cavity, lungs, intestine, nerves, muscles, vagina, kidneys, and marrow function.

A combination of corticosteroids and immunosuppressive agents are used to treat GVHD. Antimicrobial prophylaxis is an important aspect of treatment.

Other Late Complications

- Cataracts
- Cystitis, nephropathy, late renal failure
- Dental decay
- Chronic pulmonary problems
- Gonadal dysfunction
- Thyroid dysfunction
- Avascular necrosis of the bone
- Second malignancies
- Impaired memory and learning disorders
- Late graft failure

Supportive Management

Nutritional support remains an essential aspect of patient care throughout the transplant process. Pain management must not be overlooked in this population. Support groups for patients and family members can be helpful.

Physical and psychological follow-up is warranted in caring for the donor.

Chapter 13

Biotherapy

Biotherapy is the use of agents derived from biological sources or that affect biologic responses. Biological agents have gained acceptance as standard therapy in oncology and are used for primary or supportive care in solid tumors and hematological malignancies and in the bone marrow setting. Recombinant DNA technology allowed the production of these agents. Biological agents include those that

- restore, augment, or modulate the host's immunological mechanism,
- have direct antitumor activity, and
- have other biological effects.

Hematopoietic Growth Factors

One of the most successful applications of biotherapy has been the use of hematopoietic growth factors (HGFs) as supportive therapy for myelosuppressive chemotherapy or bone marrow transplantation (BMT). HGFs are cytokines, hormones, colony-stimulating factors, and other molecules that influence the development of bone marrow cells.

Food and Drug Administration–HGF include those listed in Table 13.1.

Anticancer Cytokine Therapy

Interferon

Interferons (IFNs) are being used as biotherapy in low- and high-dose regimens and in combination with other cytokines and chemotherapy regimens. The types of IFNs, function, and indications are listed in Table 13.2.

PART III

Table 13.1 FDA-Approved Hematopoietic Growth Factors			
Agent	Generic Name	Trade Name	Indication
Granulocyte–colony-stimulating factor (G-CSF)	Filgrastim	Neupogen (Amgen)	Decreases neutropenia
Granulocyte–macrophage-colony stimulating factor (GM-CSF)	Sargramostim	Leukine (Immunex)	Accelerates bone marrow recovery after BMT
Erythropoietin alfa	Epoietin alfa	Procrit (Ortho-Biotech, Inc.) Epogen (Amgen, Inc.)	Treatment of anemia in patients on chemotherapy
Interleukin-11	Oprelvekin	Neumega (Genetics Institute)	Prevents thrombocytopenia following myelosuppressive chemotherapy

Toxicities depend on type of IFN, dose, and schedule. Typical side effects

- *Acute*
  - Fever, chills, rigor
  - Malaise
  - Myalgia
  - Headache
  - Nausea, vomiting, diarrhea
- *Chronic*
  - Anorexia, weight loss
  - Fatigue
  - Mental slowing, confusion
  - Neutropenia, thrombocytopenia
  - Increased liver enzymes

Interleukins
Interleukins (ILs) are cytokines that act primarily between lymphocytes, and act as messengers to

Table 13.2   Types of IFNs Functions and Indications

Type/ Subtype	Function	Commercial Product	Indications
Type I			
IFN-a	Antiviral; antiproliferative	IFN alfa 2A Roferon (Roche)	Chronic hepatitis C, Chronic myelogenous leukemia, Hairy cell leukemia, AIDS-related Kaposi's sarcoma
	Antiviral; antiproliferative	IFN alfa 2B Intron A (Schering)	Hairy cell leukemia, AIDS-related Kaposi's sarcoma, Chronic hepatitis B, Adjuvant therapy for follicular lymphoma and melanoma
		Infergen (Amgen)	Hepatitis C
IFN-b	Antiviral	IFN beta 1b and 1a	Multiple sclerosis
Type II			
IFN-g	Immunomodulatory	IFN gamma 1b Actimmune (Genentech)	Chronic granulomatous disease

PART III

initiate, coordinate, and amplify immune defense activities.

Interleukin-2

Stimulates cytotoxic lymphoid cells, natural killer (NK) cells, lymphokine-activated killer (LAK) cells, B cells, complement factors, monocytes, and macrophages. IL-2 is approved for the treatment of renal cell carcinoma and malignant melanoma.

Toxicities are dose-dependent and include the following:

- General (flulike): Fever, chills, and rigors occur within 2 to 8 hours of drug administration, and symptoms are most severe after initial doses.
- Gastrointestinal: nausea, vomiting, diarrhea, anorexia, taste changes, stomatitis
- Dermatologic: pruritic, macular erythematous rash progressing to dry desquamation; peeling skin on palms and soles
- Neurologic: confusion, hallucination, agitation, cognitive changes, depression, sleep disturbances
- Cardiovascular/pulmonary: hypotension, tachycardia, arrhythmias, fluid retention, edema, weight gain, dyspnea; partially related to capillary leak syndrome
- Renal: increased creatinine and blood urea nitrogen, oliguria, azotemia
- Hepatic: elevated SGOT, SGPT, LDH, alkaline phosphatase and bilirubin; jaundice and hepatomegaly
- Hematologic: anemia, thrombocytopenia, leukopenia, eosinophilia, and impaired neutrophil function

Interleukin-1
Primary coordinator of the body's inflammatory response to microbial invasion. No significant tumor responses have been reported. Side effects include fever, rigors, nausea, and dose-limiting hypotension.

Interleukin-4, Interleukin-6, and Interleukin-12
Clinical trials have shown limited response.

Tumor Necrosis Factors
Produced by macrophages, NK cells, and T cells, which cause a variety of immune response ac-

tions. To date, tumor necrosis factor has not received regulatory approval.

Monoclonal Antibodies

Monoclonal antibodies (MAbs) are artificially produced antibodies and have three essential roles in cancer therapy:

1. Diagnostic and screening functions
2. Purging autologous bone marrow of malignant cells ex vivo
3. Cancer therapy capable of killing tumor cells

The side effects of MAbs depend on the agent used. However, acute infusion-related allergic reactions are common because some or all of the MAb consists of foreign proteins. Symptoms (fever, chills, rigors, nausea and vomiting, fatigue, headache, rhinitis, and more severe hypersensitivity reactions) usually begin within 30 minutes to 2 hours after the start of the first infusion.

Approved Therapeutic Monoclonal Antibodies

- Rituximab (Rituxin , Genentech): treatment of relapsed or refactory low-grade or follicular CD20-positive B-cell non-Hodgkin's lymphoma
- Trastuzumab (Herceptin, Genentech): treatment of patients with metastatic breast cancer whose tumors overexpress the HER2 protein

Other Immunomodulating Agents

These agents stimulate host defense mechanisms or augment immunity. Agents approved for cancer therapy or clinical trials include the following:

- Bacillus Calmette-Guørin (BCG): FDA approved as intravesical treatment of carcinoma of the bladder; also used as intralesional injection for melanoma lesions
- Retinoids: Tretinoin is indicated for treatment of acute promyelocytic leukemia; other

retinoids have shown activity in chemoprevention trials.

Cancer Vaccines

Vaccine therapy involves the administration of antigens to stimulate the patient's immune system. Although clinical trials have not shown significant improvement with vaccine therapy, clinical data with melanoma vaccines are encouraging.

Nursing Management

Biological agents are reconstituted predominantly by nurses and patients. Patients commonly self-inject these agents. Biotherapy has a distinctive constellation of side effects.

Flulike Syndrome

- Evaluate the risk for flulike syndrome (FLS) symptoms: Cytokines, monoclonal antibody infusions, and the first dose of IFNs are the highest risk factors.
- Premedicate with acetaminophen or indomethacin 1 hour prior to the first dose of biological therapy.
- Use warm blankets at the first sign of a chill.
- For rigors, administer meperidine 25 to 50 mg parenterally as appropriate.
- For arthralgia, myalgia, or headache, continue acetaminophen as appropriate.

Fatigue

- Assess peak severity, patterns of activity and sleep, and the impact on self-care activities and nutritional balance.
- Teach the patient and family methods of saving energy and the value of activity in spite of fatigue.
- Encourage the patient to maintain activity and avoid prolonged bed rest.

Cardiovascular and Respiratory Changes
- Assess the patient's status at frequent intervals during high-dose IL-2 therapy.
- Evaluate left ventricular function in all patients prior to and during treatment with trastuzumab.
- Teach the patient to report chest pain, edema, palpitations, or changes in respiration.

Capillary Leak Syndrome
- Monitor blood pressure, pulse, respiratory status, urine output, and body weight during therapy.
- Remove all jewelry, particularly rings, before treatment.
- For hypotension and oliguria, administer fluid boluses. Low-dose dopamine may be administered intravenously to increase urine output.
- Instruct the patient to report any feelings of dizziness.

Dermatological Changes
- Frequently apply hypoallergenic emollient lotions and creams on the patient's skin.
- For pruritus, administer antipruritic medications such as hydroxyzine HCL or diphenhydramine. Use lorazepam with severe itching as needed. Try colloidal oatmeal baths.
- For subcutaneous site inflammation, rotate the sites and do not reuse them until firmness resolves.

Gastrointestinal Symptoms
- Steroids should not be used as an antiemetic because of their effects on immune function.
- Administer antiemetics and antidiarrheal agents as needed.
- Monitor for fluid and electrolyte imbalance.

Neurological Effects
- Assess baseline neurological function.

PART III

- Instruct family members on the early signs of mental status changes that should be reported to the patient's health team.
- Monitor the patient throughout therapy, because symptoms, especially mental status changes, can be subtle.

Anaphylactic Reactions

- Have essential drugs, steroids, epinephrine, and antihistamines available when administering MAb therapy or for patients with a history of hypersensitivity reactions.
- Follow manufacturer's guidelines regarding the infusion-related symptom complex.

Chapter 14

......

Gene Therapy

Gene therapy involves the transferring of corrected or altered genes into a person's cells, and therefore has the potential to cure or improve health conditions. One hundred thousand genes reside in each individual's human genome. Genes are made of a chemical code (DNA) particular to each gene. The code directs the composition and production of proteins that make up living tissue and regulates all of the body's functions.

Genetic disorders arise when an error in the multistep process of replication and cell division occurs. The error may lead to disability or even death. Three types of genetic alterations involve gene therapy:

1. Single gene (e.g., Mendelian genetic disorders)
2. Multifactorial (e.g., heart disease, high blood pressure, cancer, mental illness)
3. Acquired genetic conditions (e.g., viral infections such as hepatitis or AIDs)

Principles and Goals of Gene Therapy

The application of gene therapy includes the following:

- *Somatic gene therapy* directed at the somatic cells, the nonreproductive cells of the body, and intended to correct inherited genetic disorders
- *Germ-line gene therapy* aimed at altering sperm and ova
- *Enhancement gene therapy*, which is the placement of genes in an embryo or offspring that would improve a societal desirable trait

Successful gene therapy requires efficient gene delivery to human cells. Gene transfer methods include the following:

- Recombinant virus vectors
- Chemical methods
- Physical methods
- Fusion methods
- Receptor-mediated endocytosis

Vectors for Gene Transfer

Current gene therapy uses viral vectors to deliver the therapeutic gene. Effective gene therapy requires the following:

- Efficient delivery of the gene to the target tissue
- Sustaining long-term gene expression
- Assurance that the gene transfer will not harm the patient
- Assurance that the corrected gene is transferred to nondividing cells

Viral Vectors

A variety of vector systems to transfer the gene have been developed:

- Retrovirus composed of RNA that can insert itself into dividing cells
- Adenovirus composed of DNA that does not integrate into host DNA and require actively dividing cells to introduce their therapeutic gene
- Adeno-associated virus, composed of a single strand of DNA, which can infect a variety of types of cells and shows promise as a potential vector for in vivo gene therapy
- Herpes virus, which infects cells of the nervous system and may be a useful vector for gene therapy

Nonviral Vectors

These methods may be easier to manufacture and safer. To integrate into the human genome, nonviral methods rely on transfer of therapeutic genes into human cells by chemical methods and encapsulation of therapeutic genes into liposomes.

Clinical Protocols for Gene Therapy

Treatment of cancer using gene therapy aims to inhibit oncogene function and restore tumor-suppressor function. Oncogenes stimulate neoplastic growth. Antioncogenes (or tumor-suppressor genes) block the action of growth-inducing proteins. When functioning normally, tumor-suppressor genes and proto-oncogenes enable the body to perform vital functions, such as replacing dead cells and repairing defective ones.

Clinical gene therapy trials include

- gene-marking protocols,
- gene therapy protocols, and
- nonviral gene therapy protocols.

Ethical, Social, and Legal Issues

Ethical issues regarding gene therapy are a major societal concern. Ethical guidelines include

- concern for the clinical benefit of all persons receiving gene therapy,
- assurance of informed consent,
- fair selection of persons for gene therapy research protocols,
- attention to the need for biosafety protocols,
- public involvement in genetic research policy, and
- attention to long-term consequences of genetic research.

Practice Implications for Oncology Nurses

The evolution of genetics is leading to continuous changes in nursing practice. Nursing responsibilities include the following:

- *Direct care:* educate patients, administer gene therapy, and monitor and manage side effects

- *Educator:* provide information to patient, family, and public
- *Advocate:* assure privacy and confidentiality of genetic information and protect against discrimination
- *Genetics services provider:* gather family history and identify need of further genetic education
- *Research investigator:* participate in clinical research trials

Chapter 15
··············

Late Effects of Cancer Treatment

Scope of the Problem
Long-term, disease-free survival from pediatric and adult cancers continues to improve. It is projected that by 2010, one in every 250 young adults between 15 to 45 years of age will be a survivor of childhood cancer.

The late effects of cancer result from the physiological effects of particular treatments or the interactions among treatment, the disease, and the individual. Late effects, or the expression of tissue damage, can appear months to years after treatment. The effects can be mild to severe to life-threatening.

Central Nervous System
Late effects as a result of central nervous system (CNS) treatment have been observed in survivors of acute lymphocytic leukemia (ALL) and brain tumors, and after bone marrow transplantation.

Neuropsychological Late Effects
- Declines in general intellectual abilities and deficits in visual-motor skills, attention, memory, and verbal fluency are the most frequent late effects.
- Associated with cranial radiation alone or in combination with intrathecal (IT) chemotherapy.
- Progress over time and become observable as cognitive abilities begin to lag behind age.

Neuroanatomical Changes
- Brain atrophy, leukoencephalopathy, and white matter changes have been found in 50% of chil-

dren with ALL who received high-dose methotrexate or IT methotrexate and cranial radiation.

Vision and Hearing

- Cataracts and retinopathy are associated with radiation therapy.
- Conjunctivitis, keratitis, retinal hemorrhage, retinopathy, optic neuritis, and blurred vision are common ocular toxicities due to chemotherapy.
- Hearing loss is closely associated with cisplatin therapy.

Immune System

Some aspects of immune function can remain impaired for years after treatment.

Cardiovascular System

Cardiac toxicity, presenting as cardiomyopathy with signs of congestive heart failure, is the most serious late effect of the anthracyclines.

Delayed radiation injury to the heart (e.g., mediastinal radiation) can manifest as pericardial, myocardial, or coronary heart disease.

Pulmonary System

Pneumonitis and pulmonary fibrosis are major late effects due to bleomycin, alkylating agents, and radiation therapy.

Gastrointestinal System

Radiation and radiation-enhancing chemotherapeutic agents have long-term effects on the gastrointestinal tract and liver:

- Esophageal and gastric ulceration
- Intestinal injury following pelvic radiation usually appears 2 to 5 years after treatment. The injury can manifest as diarrhea, bleeding, pain, fistula formation, and obstruction.

- Hepatic fibrosis, cirrhosis, and portal hypertension are common late effects in the liver.

Renal System

Nephritis and cystitis are long-term renal toxicities documented in patients treated with cyclophosphamide, ifosfamide, and cisplatin. Radiation also can damage the kidneys.

Endocrine System

Cancer treatment can cause adverse effects in a number of endocrine functions.

Thyroid

- Hypothyroidism is a result of >2000 cGy radiation or >750 cGy total body irradiation.
- Hypothyroidism usually develops 3 to 4 years after treatment but can occur as late as 7 to 14 years later.
- Young children, tumors of head and neck, brain tumors, lymphomas, leukemia with cranial radiation, and bone marrow transplant patients are high-risk factors.

Hypothalamic–Pituitary Axis

- Growth impairment and short stature occur with CNS radiation.
- Doses greater than 2400 cGy result in hypothalamic dysfunction.
- Doses greater than 4000 cGy result in pituitary dysfunction.
- Patients at high risk include those with leukemia with CNS radiation, CNS tumors, and head and neck tumors.

Ovaries

- Permanent damage to gonads can result from chemotherapy (e.g., cyclophosphamide, ifosfamide, busulfan, mechlorethamine, procarbazine) and 400 to 1000 cGy radiation (age dependent).

- Primary ovarian failure with amenorrhea, decreased estradiol, and elevated hormone levels occurs in women who have received alkylating agents.
- Younger females fail to develop secondary sexual characteristics or have arrested pubertal development.
- The risk population includes women over 40 years of age and those with abdominal and pelvic tumors, Hodgkin's disease, and spinal radiation.
- Decreased libido and dyspareunia affect sexual function.

Testes
- Decreased or absent spermatogonia can occur in males treated with alkylating agents.
- The testes are very sensitive to radiation.
  - More than 600 cGy leads to permanent azoospermia.
  - More than 2400 cGy causes Leydig cell damage and decreased testosterone.
- The risk population includes patients with lymphomas, pelvic tumor, testicular tumors, and leukemia with testicular infiltrates.
- Erectile dysfunction and decreased libido result in sexual dysfunction.

Musculoskeletal System
Children treated before 6 years of age or those in puberty are at highest risk for musculoskeletal changes. Most late effects of this system are associated with radiation:

- Scoliosis, kyphosis, or both, due to radiation to one side of the body
- Spinal shortening
- Functional limitations, shortening, osteonecrosis, avascular necrosis of the long bones

- Altered growth of facial bones, dental problems, and facial asymmetry following maxillo-facial or orbital radiation
- Skin changes and lymphedema

Surgical procedures such as amputation or limb disarticulation have many long-term effects.

Fatigue

Survivors of bone marrow transplant report fatigue up to 18 years posttreatment. Breast cancer survivors have reported fatigue 2 to 10 years after treatment. Children experience fatigue for many years after radiation therapy.

Second Malignant Neoplasms

Acute nonlymphocytic leukemia is the most common chemotherapy-related second malignancy resulting from the use of alkylating agents. It occurs 5 to 10 years after treatment.

Sarcomas of the bone and soft tissue are the most common second malignant neoplasm after radiation therapy. The incidence of sarcomas ranges from 10 to 20 years after treatment.

Early Detection and Prevention

Survivors of cancer require life-long follow-up care. Drugs that minimize toxicities are undergoing development and testing.

PART III

Chapter 16

• • • • • • • • • • • • • •

Alternative Methods and Complementary Therapies in Cancer Management

Each year, more than half of the million Americans diagnosed with cancer are cured with scientifically sound therapies. Each year, thousands of cancer patients use alternative cancer remedies to prevent, diagnose, or treat cancer. The American Cancer Society provides the following definitions:

- *Alternative therapies* are unproven or disproven methods that are used in the place of mainstream, or conventional, treatment.
- *Complementary therapies* are supportive therapies that are used to complement standard conventional therapy.

The National Center for Complementary and Alternative Medicine (NCCAM) supports clinical research centers in conducting research on complementary and alternative medicine therapies. Oncology nurses are involved with complementary therapies that are proven adjuncts in the care of cancer patients.

Who Seeks Alternative and Complementary Cancer Treatments
Limited studies report that patients who seek such therapies are

- white,
- educated,

- higher socioeconomic status, and
- interested in a greater sense of self-control.

Popular Alternative and Complementary Methods

Diet and Nutrition

Alternative cancer treatments involving diet often promote that foods or food supplements can cure cancer. There are many different types of metabolic regimens. Metabolic therapy is the manipulation of diet and detoxification by enemas to remove toxins from the body. Popular methods include

- the Gerson regimen (strict diet, purgatives, and enemas),
- macrobiotic diets (cancer preventive effects under study), and
- megavitamins (megadoses of vitamin C can cause kidney damage).

Pharmacological and Biological Approaches

These therapies are highly controversial. Popular treatments include

- antineoplaston therapy,
- immunoaugmentative therapy,
- Cancell (a formula of chemicals that supposedly reacts with the body electrically and lowers the voltage of a cancer cell),
- dimethyl sulfoxide,
- live-cell therapy (injection of cells from animals),
- oxymedicine (hydrogen peroxide, ozone gas administered orally, rectally, intravenously, intramuscularly, and vaginally), and
- shark cartilage.

Mind–Body Techniques

Popular complementary methods can help patients feel better and improve their quality of life.

PART III

However, these techniques must not be promoted as cancer cures. Helpful complementary approaches include:

- Aromatherapy
- Art therapy
- Biofeedback
- Herbals (ginger tea for nausea or heartburn; chamomile tea for indigestion; valerian tea for sleep problems)
- Massage therapy
- Meditation
- Music therapy
- Physical activity
- Prayer, spiritual practices
- Support groups
- Tai chi
- Yoga

Herbal Remedies
- Essiac tea (studies have shown no benefit)
- Pau d'arco tea (active ingredient can be harmful to humans)
- Iscador (popular in Europe)
- Chaparral tea (can cause liver damage and failure)

Alternative Medical Systems
Chinese medicine and India's Ayurvedic medicine are popular.

Manual Healing Methods
Therapeutic touch (no direct touch) and manipulation techniques have been promoted as manual healing. Hands-on massage, to reduce stress, is a useful complementary therapy for some patients.

Bioelectromagnetics
These therapies use electromagnetic low frequency to penetrate the body and heal damaged tissues.

Practitioners of Alternative Methods

Promoters rely on testimonials and anecdotes. There is a lack of scientific evidence as to the effectiveness of these methods. Tijuana, Mexico, is a haven for alternative treatment facilities.

Safety and Efficacy

Any new method of cancer treatment in the United States must meet certain scientific standards before it receives government approval for interstate distribution. State governments also participate in regulation. Organizations provide information to health professionals and the public about alternative methods, and these sources include the following:

- American Cancer Society: (800)ACS-2345, or http://www.cancer.org
- University of Texas Center for Alternative Medicine Research in Cancer: http://www.sph.uth.tmc.edu/utcam/default .htm
- NIH Center for Complementary and Alternative Medicine: http://altmed.od.nih.gov/
- Cancer guide by Steve Dunn: http://cancerguide.org
- National Council for Reliable Information: http://www.ncahf.org
- Quackwatch: http://www.quackwatch.com
- American Botanical Council: http://www.herbalgram.org
- U.S. Pharmacopoeia Consumer Information: http://www.usp.org

PART III

Role of Nurses and Nursing Interventions

Be knowledgeable of alternative and complementary therapies, the risks of such methods, and toxicity if the patient is using them in combination with standard therapy.

Assess communication channels and patient motivations for potential use.

Maintain positive communication channels with the patient and family who may be interested in or participating in such methods.

Many patients turn to alternative methods because they do not feel like a participant in their care, so it is important that patients and family participate in the health care process.

Part IV

Symptom Management

Chapter 17

Bleeding Disorders

Scope of the Problem

Bleeding is one of the most serious, potentially life-threatening problems for the person with cancer. Multiple hemostatic abnormalities may be involved in cancer-associated bleeding. Minor bleeding may be a presenting symptom of cancer. Severe bleeding may indicate progressive cancer.

Physiological Alterations

Causes of bleeding in cancer are primarily due to platelet abnormalities or coagulation abnormalities.

Platelet Abnormalities

Thrombocytopenia, a reduction in platelets, is the most frequent platelet abnormality and is often due to the following:

- Decreased platelet production due to tumor invasion of the bone marrow or to acute or delayed effects of chemotherapy or radiation therapy
- Abnormal platelet distribution due to hypersplenism: 90% of platelet production may be sequestered in the spleen and unavailable in circulation
- Platelet destruction or dysfunction as a result of cancer or immune-mediated thrombocytopenia. Often, drugs such as aspirin, nonsteroidal antiinflammatory agents, and antibiotics destroy platelets and prolong bleeding time.
- Platelet dilution due to multiple transfusions
- Disseminated intravascular coagulation (DIC) due to infection, tumor, liver disease, or intravascular hemorrhage

Thrombocythemia/thrombocytosis occurs due to the overproduction of platelets. Bleeding and thrombosis are common.

Coagulation Abnormalities
Hypocoagulation is often due to

- liver disease,
- deficiency of vitamin K, and
- excessive frozen plasma transfusions post-surgery.

Bleeding tends to occur in deep areas of the body or into the joint.

Clinical Manifestations
Risk of spontaneous hemorrhage is considered to be greater than 50% when the platelet count is less that 20,000 cells/mm^3. Manifestations of a low platelet count include

- easy bruising,
- petechiae,
- ecchymosis,
- melena,
- hematuria, and
- bleeding from the gums, nose, and mouth.

Assessment
Patient/Family History
- Bleeding tendencies
- Signs or symptoms of anemia
- Medication history (chemotherapy or other drugs that may affect platelets)
- Acute bacterial or viral infections that may increase risk for DIC
- General performance status
- Transfusion history
- Nutritional status (vitamin K or vitamin C deficiency)
- Immunological disorders such as idiopathic thrombocytopenic purpura (ITP)

Physical Examination

Central Nervous System

- Mental status changes, confusion
- Lethargy, restlessness
- Changes in cognition or level of consciousness
- Obtundation, seizures, coma
- Changes in neurological signs, including widening in pulse pressure, pupil size and reactivity, motor strength and coordination, speech and paralysis, or headache

Eyes and Ears

- Visual disturbances, including diplopia, blurred vision, and partial field loss
- Increased injection on the sclera, periorbital edema, and subconjunctival hemorrhage
- Headache
- Eye or ear pain

Nose, Mouth, and Throat

- Petechiae on nasal and/or oral mucosa
- Ulcerations
- Gingival or mucous membrane bleeding
- Epistaxis

Cardiovascular

- Changes in vital signs, color, and temperature of all extremities
- Abnormal peripheral pulses
- Tachycardia
- Hypotension
- Angina

Pulmonary

- Dyspnea, tachypnea, and shortness of breath
- Crackles, wheezes, stridor, and orthopnea
- Hemoptysis and cyanosis

Abdominal

- Pain in right upper quadrant with abdominal distention may be indicative of hepatomegaly.

- Left flank or shoulder pain may be indicative of splenomegaly.
- Vague abdominal pain may be indicative of retroperitoneal bleeding.
- Blood around the rectum, tarry stools, and frank or occult blood in stools
- Hematemesis

Genitourinary System
- Blood in the urine
- Dysuria, burning, frequency, and pain on urination
- Need for assessment of character and amount of menses
- Decreased urine output may be due to acute tubular necrosis or hypovolemia and shock.

Musculoskeletal System
- Warm, tender, swollen joints with diminished mobility for active and passive range of motion may indicate bleeding into the joints.

Integumentary System
- Bruising, petechiae, and purpura
- Ecchymosis and hematomas
- Pallor
- Jaundice
- Oozing from venipuncture sites or injections, biopsy sites, central line catheters, or nasogastric tubes

PART IV

Screening Tests
- *Platelet count* below 100,000 cells/mm^3 is considered indicative of thrombocytopenia. Below 15,000 cells/mm^3 presents risk for spontaneous hemorrhage. Above 400,000 cells/mm^3 presents risk for thrombocytosis.
- *Bleeding time* measures the time it takes for a small skin incision to stop bleeding. The normal range is 1 to 9 minutes.

- *Whole-blood retraction* test measures the speed and extent of blood clot retraction in a test tube. A normal clot shrinks to half its size in 1 to 2 hours.
- *Bone marrow aspirate* will usually reveal the etiology of thrombocytopenia.
- *Activated partial thromboplastin time* (aPTT) screens for coagulation deficiencies. There is a risk for spontaneous bleeding if the aPTT is greater than 100.
- *Prothrombin time* (PT) screens for coagulation deficiencies. Prolonged PT values are seen in liver disease and with coumarin therapy.
- *International normalized ratio* (INR) is a measure of coagulation and is usually less than 2.0. An INR greater than 2.0 is considered anticoagulated.
- *Fibrin degradation products* test for fibrinolysis, as seen in DIC and primary fibrinolytic disorders.

Treatment

General Prevention
Bleeding precautions are instituted for any patient at risk of bleeding. Preventive measures include the following:

- Apply direct and steady pressure to site of bleeding. Apply cold compresses.
- Avoid intramuscular or subcutaneous injections.
- Prevent forceful coughing, sneezing, nose blowing, or vomiting.
- Provide for liberal use of stool softeners and laxatives.
- Colony-stimulating growth factors (e.g., interleukin-11, erythropoietin) may accelerate hematological recovery.
- Cytoprotectant agents such as amifostine may protect against treatment-associated thrombocytopenia.

Managemant of Bleeding

Thrombocytopenia

- Determine the underlying cause.
- Treat the primary disease.
- Give platelet transfusions.
- Adjust the chemotherapy dose or schedule.
- Provide steroid therapy or splenectomy for the mangement of ITP.

Hypocoagulation

- Effective tumor therapy
- Plasma and plasma derivative therapy
- Albumin transfusions
- Plasma component therapy
- Parenteral vitamin K

Blood Component Therapy

Red Blood Cell Therapy

- This therapy for anemia is indicated to treat decreased red cell production secondary to myelosuppressive therapy and/or the primary disease process.
- Transfusions are indicated when the patient is short of breath.
- Transfusion of 1 unit of red blood cells increases the hematocrit by 3% or the hemoglobin concentration by 1 g/dL in a 70-kg nonbleeding patient.
- Packed red blood cells provide more than 70% of the hematocrit of whole blood with one-third the plasma.
- Leukocyte-reduced blood component therapy minimizes antigenic reactions.
- All blood products given to a severely immunocompromised host should be irradiated to prevent lymphocyte engraftment.

Platelet Therapy

- Platelet transfusions are required when the patient is at risk for bleeding or when bleeding occurs in patients with a low platelet count.

- One unit of platelets increases peripheral blood platelet level by 10,000 to 12,000 cells/mm^3.
- The goal is to maintain a platelet count above 15,000 to 20,000 cells/mm^3 to prevent spontaneous bleeding.
- Platelets are generally not transfused for ITP because doing so is rarely effective.
- Failure to maintain an adequate platelet count often results from infection, fever, DIC, or splenomegaly.
- Fever caused by platelets may be prevented by premedicating with antipyretics, corticosteroids, and/or antihistamines; meperidine may be given if the patient is having shaking chills.
- Repeated exposure to human leukocyte antigens (HLAs) on donor platelets may result in ineffective platelet therapy, requiring HLA-matched or single-donor platelet transfusions.

Plasma Therapy
- Plasma component therapy is used to treat coagulation disorders, shock, severe bleeding, bleeding associated with infections, and management of acute DIC.

Transfusion Complications
There are many risks associated with blood component therapy. Transfusion reactions can be immediate or delayed.

Immediate Blood Transfusion Reactions
- Transfusion of ABO-incompatible blood
- Circulatory overload with respiratory distress
- Air embolism
- Hypothermia
- Bacterial contamination of blood

- Reactions are seen most frequently in recipients of multiple transfusions.
- Treatment consists of acetaminophen for the fever, meperidine for severe rigors, and steroids for dyspnea.
- Allergic reactions account for about 1% of transfusion reactions.
- Allergic reactions may be severe, manifested by bronchospasm, laryngeal edema, and anaphylaxis.

Delayed Blood Transfusion Reactions
- Graft-versus-host disease (GVHD) is a delayed transfusion reaction in patients who are severely immunosuppressed. The donor competent T lymphocyte immunologically attacks the immunocompromised host tissue after transfusion.
- Posttransfusion GVHD is fatal almost 90% of the time.
- Patients at risk include bone marrow transplant recipients, peripheral blood stem cell recipients, patients undergoing combination treatment for Hodgkin's and non-Hodgkin's lymphoma, and leukemia patients undergoing induction chemotherapy.
- To prevent posttransfusion GVHD, all blood products given to severely immunocompromised patients are irradiated with at least 2500 cGY to prevent proliferation of lymphocytes.

Home Transfusion Therapy
Basic selection criteria
- Cooperative patient
- Stable cardiopulmonary status of the patient
- Physical limitations that make transportation difficult
- Absence of reactions to the most recent blood transfusion

PART IV

- A diagnosis supporting the need for blood transfusion therapy
- Patients who do not have an acute need for blood or who do not require more than 2 units in a 24-hour period
- Access to a telephone for medical needs
- Having a responsible adult home during and after the blood transfusion

Chapter 18

......

Fatigue

Scope of the Problem

Fatigue is one of the most common and distressing symptoms associated with the diagnosis and treatment of cancer, and it has a major impact on all aspects of a patient's life. Fatigue affects the majority of patients with cancer and may last for years after treatment has been completed. Fatigue has been described as an overwhelming sense of exhaustion, tiredness, and a decreased capacity for physical and mental work.

Etiology and Risk Factors

Although the exact cause of fatigue is unknown, it is considered to be related to the following factors:

- Physiological factors (e.g., anemia, pain, fever, surgery, radiation therapy, chemotherapy, and biological response modifiers)
- Psychological and situational factors (e.g., anxiety, depression, sleep disturbances, immobility, and decreased activity)

Clinical Manifestations

The manifestations of fatigue can be subjective or objective. Subjective manifestations relate to the individual's perception:

- Emotional or psychological and physical feelings
- Perception of interference with activities of daily living
- Amount of distress

Objective manifestations can be assessed by another; for example:

- Weight loss

- Anemia
- Decreased energy
- Apathy
- Decreased attention
- Changes in sleep patterns

Assessment

The initial assessment should include the following:

- Pattern, onset, duration, and intensity of fatigue
- A complete history
- Exploration of the patient's perceptions, factors that increase or alleviate fatigue, sleep patterns, lifestyle, concentration level, and nutritional intake
- A complete physical examination, with diagnostic and laboratory tests for anemia and other physiological causes

It is helpful to have the patient keep a diary of the occurrence and level of fatigue. A numerical or visual analog scale is useful.

Treatment

Before treatment is begun, information about fatigue and the likelihood of its occurrence will help the patient more easily cope and develop self-care behaviors. Nursing management of fatigue involves instruction for self-care activities, such as conservation of energy, exercise, rest and sleep, and motivational strategies, and the treatment of anemia.

Energy Conservation

- Limit energy expenditure.
- Prioritize and rearrange activities.
- Decrease nonessential activities.
- Increase dependence on others for home management.
- Develop energy-saving ideas.

Exercise
- Follow an individualized plan of exercise.
- Do nonstrenuous exercise (e.g., walking, stretching, or yoga).

Rest and Sleep
- Space rest periods with activity or exercise.
- Avoid caffeine and alcohol.
- Establish a regular bedtime.
- Establish a quiet environment.
- Take a warm bath; sip warm milk or herbal teas.
- Use relaxation techniques.

Motivation
- Encourage verbalization of thoughts and feelings.
- Emphasize the positive aspects of life.
- Encourage participation and control in the treatment plan.
- Encourage communication with friends and loved ones.

Treatment of Anemia
- Carefully assess and monitor the patient if anemia is present.
- Use of erythropoietin is effective treatment for anemia, and is associated with enhanced quality of life.
- Monitor patients receiving transfusions or erythropoietin.

Chapter 19
∙∙∙∙∙∙∙∙∙∙∙∙∙∙

Hypercalcemia

Scope of the Problem
Hypercalcemia is the most common metabolic complication of malignancy and can be life-threatening. Approximately 10% to 40% of cancer patients experience hypercalcemia as a late complication of cancer. Hypercalcemia occurs most frequently in patients with breast cancer, lung cancer, and multiple myeloma. Incidence, however, may be decreasing due to the widespread use of bisphosphonates.

Hyperparathyroidism is the most frequent cause of hypercalcemia and generally develops over a long period of time. Cancer-induced hypercalcemia most often develops rapidly, necessitating prompt diagnosis and treatment. Other causes of hypercalcemia include hormone manipulation, vitamin D intoxication, or other idiopathic causes.

Hypercalcemia of Malignancy
Hypercalcemia occurs when more calcium is resorbed from bone than is deposited in bone. There are two primary causes of hypercalcemia: humoral hypercalcemia of malignancy (HHM) or local osteolytic hypercalcemia (LOH).

Humoral Hypercalcemia of Malignancy
HHM causes 80% of cases. Patients may or may not have bone metastases but often have tumors that secrete hormones and cytokines that cause calcium resorption from bone and hypercalcemia.

Local Osteolytic Hypercalcemia
LOH occurs primarily in patients with extensive osteolytic bone metastases. Tumor cells do not re-

sorb bone but produce factors that induce local bone absorption, osteolysis, and hypercalcemia. Local production of parathyroid hormone–related peptide by tumor cells enhances tumor growth in the bone.

Pathophysiology

The majority (99%) of the total calcium of the body is bound in bones and teeth. Only 1% of calcium is found in the serum and the majority is ionized calcium, which is filtered in the kidney. The kidney regulates and maintains serum calcium levels in a constant narrow range.

- Women: 8.9 to 10.2 mg/dL
- Men: 9.0 to 10.3 mg/dL
- Hypercalcemia is diagnosed when the serum calcium exceeds 11.0 mg/dL.

Clinical Manifestations

Individuals who develop hypercalcemia may be asymptomatic or have a number of signs and symptoms that may be misinterpreted as terminal cancer or side effects of treatment. There is little relation between symptoms and calcium level.

Neurologic

Central nervous system

- Impaired concentration
- Confusion
- Apathy
- Drowsiness or lethargy
- Late: obtundation, coma

Peripheral neuromuscular

- Muscle weakness
- Hypotonia
- Decreased or absent deep-tendon reflexes

Gastrointestinal
- Increased gastric acid secretion
- Nausea, vomiting, and anorexia
- Constipation

Renal
- Polyuria
- Polydipsia
- Dehydration (thirst, dry mucosa, decreased or absent perspiration, poor skin turgor, and concentrated urine)

Cardiovascular
- Slow cardiac conduction (prolonged P-R interval, widened QRS, shortened QT, ST intervals)
- Bradycardia (with rapid increases)
- Bradyarrhythmias can progress to bundle branch block, atrioventricular block with complete heart block or asystole.

Assessment and Grading
The diagnostic work-up includes a history, physical examination, and laboratory tests.

Hypercalcemia may be graded as follows:
- Mild hypercalcemia: >10.3 to <12 mg/dL
- Moderate hypercalcemia: 12 to 14 mg/dL
- Severe hypercalcemia: 14 to 16 mg/dL
- Life-threatening hypercalcemia: >16 mg/dL

These values assume a normal serum albumin. When serum albumin is less than normal, there is less albumin to bind with calcium and a formula must be used to adjust serum calcium.

Treatment
The goals of therapy are to correct dehydration, to increase renal excretion of calcium with vigorous saline diuresis, to inhibit calcium resorption from bone with antiresorptive agents, and to treat the underlying malignancy.

Saline Diuresis

- Administration of oral or intravenous saline-containing fluids is the first step to restore fluid balance and increase urinary calcium excretion.
- The rate of normal saline administration is based on severity of hypercalcemia, severity of dehydration, and cardiovascular tolerance.
- Four to 5 liters of normal saline over 24 hours results in modest decreases in serum calcium.
- A loop diuretic such as furosemide may be added after fluid balance has been restored.

Pharmacological Interventions

- *Bisphosphonates* (etidronate, pamidronate)
  - Prevent precipitation of calcium phosphate
  - Pamidronate (Aredia^{fi} 90 mg over 2 hours) is the standard drug and dosage to effectively treat hypercalcemia. Unlike etidronate, pamidronate can be safely administered to patients with impaired renal function. The adverse effects of pamidronate include mild fever and a flulike syndrome with malaise.
- *Calcitonin* may be combined with pamidronate if the patient's serum calcium is greater than 13 mg/dL.
- A *corticosteroid* may be added to enhance and prolong the effect of the calcitonin.

Other Measures

- *Prevention*: Pamidronate has been approved by the Food and Drug Administration for patients who have osteolytic bone metastases (who are not hypercalcemic) to maintain normal serum calcium levels.

PART IV

Chapter 20

Infection

Scope of the Problem

Infections are responsible for approximately 50% to 75% of cancer deaths. They may result from the underlying malignancy, intensive treatment modalities, hospitalization, or a combination of factors. *Immunocompromised host* refers to a person who has one or more defects in natural defense mechanisms that predispose to severe, sometimes life-threatening infection.

Physiological Alterations

Causes of infection in cancer patients can develop as the result of the following:

- Disruption in protective barriers (skin, mucous membranes)
- Changes in normal flora (due to antibiotic usage)
- Obstruction due to tumor
- Neutropenia
  - Individuals whose neutrophil count is less than 1,000 cells/mm^3 are considered neutropenic and are at increased risk for infection.
  - When the neutrophil count is less than 500 cells/mm^3, risk of infection is significant.
- Immunosuppression
  - Impaired immune function can be caused by viral infections and AIDS.
- Nutritional disturbance
  - Cachexia, obstruction, or direct tumor invasion of nutritional pathways can add to risk of infection.

- Cancer therapies
  - Surgery, radiation, and chemotherapy can each affect the body's defense systems and predispose to risk of infection.

Common sites of infection
- Mouth and pharynx
- Respiratory tract
- Skin and soft tissue
- Intravascular catheters
- Perineal region
- Urinary tract
- Gastrointestinal (GI) tract

Types of Infection and Specific Treatments

Bacterial Infections
Most common bacterial infections
- Gram-negative bacteria (e.g., *Escherichia coli*, *Klebsiella pneumoniae*, and *Pseudomonas aeruginosa*)
  - Primary cause of infection in granulocytopenic patients
- Gram-positive bacteria (e.g., *Staphylococcus aureus* and *Staphylococcus epidermidis*)
- Treatment is immediate empiric antibiotic therapy.
  - Highly specific therapy is initiated once an organism is identified.
  - Combination antibiotic therapy usually includes a beta-lactam antibiotic and an aminoglycoside.

Mycobacterial Infections
These infections are uncommon in cancer and are associated with defects in cellular immunity:
- Latent mycobacterial tuberculosis may reactivate.

- *Mycobacterium avium-intracellulare* (MAI) is common with AIDS.
- Treatment for mycobacterial tuberculosis is isoniazid.
- Treatment for MAI is combination antibiotic therapy.

Fungal Infections

Fungal infections are an increasingly important cause of infections for cancer patients. Factors contributing to fungal infections include the following:

- Prolonged granulocytopenia
- Implanted vascular access devices
- Administration of parenteral nutrition
- Corticosteroids
- Prolonged antibiotic therapy

Candida is the most common cause of fungal infection. *Aspergillus, Cryptococcus, Histoplasma, Phycomycetes,* and *Coccidioides* species are other fungi that cause serious infection.

Treatment is confounded by difficulty culturing the organisms and by the limited number of effective agents.

- Amphotericin B is the drug of choice.
  - Nephrotoxicity is the major side effect.
  - Side effects, including fever, chills, rigors, nausea, vomiting, hypotension, bronchospasm, and seizures, require intensive support.
- Flucytosine (5-FC), fluconazole, ketoconazole, and miconazole are also used.

Viral Infections

Most viral infections in cancer patients are caused by herpes simplex virus (HSV), varicella zoster virus (VZV), cytomegalovirus (CMV), and hepatitis A or B virus. Treatment measures include the following:

- Acyclovir is drug of choice for HSV and VZV.

- Vidarabine is effective for HSV and VZV if used early.
- Ganciclovir and foscarnet are used for CMV.

Protozoa and Parasites

Protozoal infections are associated with defects in cell-mediated immunity. They can be difficult to treat in the immunocompromised host and can quickly become life-threatening. These organisms include the following:

- *Pneumocystis carinii*
  - Fatal if untreated
  - Treat with trimethoprim-sulfamethoxazole, dapsone, or pentamidine
  - High-risk patients (e.g., AIDS patients) are sometimes treated prophylactically.
- *Toxoplasma gondii*
  - Treat with pyrimethamine plus sulfamethoxazole.
- *Cryptosporidium* (no known treatment)

Treatment

Prevention

Prevention is the most critical step in care. Simple measures include the following:

- Meticulous handwashing by caregivers
- Avoidance of crowds and infected individuals
- If granulocytopenia is present, avoidance of invasive procedures
- Adequate nutrition
- Meticulous personal hygiene
- Avoidance of skin trauma

Assessment

If the number of circulating polymorphonuclear neutrophils (PMNs) is decreased, then the host's defenses are reduced. Assessment includes key parameters:

PART IV

- Determine absolute neutrophil count (ANC). The ANC is determined by multiplying the percentage of PMNs and bands by the total number of WBCs.
  - ANC = WBC × (% PMNs + % bands)
- Culture from all potential sites of infection before giving antibiotics.

If an infection has developed, monitor the patient's response to therapy and be alert for signs of septic shock:

- Early shock
  - Low-grade fever, possible shaking chills
  - Flushed, warm skin
  - Tachycardia, normal to slightly low blood pressure
  - Transient decrease in urine output
  - Hyperventilation
  - Alert, possible mild confusion, apprehension
  - Nausea, vomiting, diarrhea
- Late shock
  - Fever
  - Cold, clammy, acrocyanosis
  - Hypotension, decreased cardiac output, peripheral edema
  - Oliguria, anuria
  - Pulmonary edema
  - Restlessness, anxiety, confusion, lethargy, coma
  - Possible blood in stool or emesis

Treatment of the Patient with Neutropenia and Fever

Ideally, a person with an infection will be treated specifically for the causative organism. With cancer patients, there are instances in which the infection develops rapidly and is so serious that empiric therapy must be initiated immediately.

Other measures to initiate immediately

- Isolation precautions and protected environment

- Administration of colony-stimulating factors (CSFs) (granulocyte and granulocyte–macrophage)
- Supportive care to maintain fluid and electrolyte levels; oxygen when needed; nutritional support

Treatment of the Patient with Gram-Negative Sepsis

Septic shock develops in 27% to 46% of cases with gram-negative bacterium. Mortality can reach 80% unless aggressive therapy is initiated.

Treatment measures to reverse shock and sepsis

- Adequate oxygenation
- Effective circulation with fluid replacement and vasoactive agents
- Immediate broad-spectrum antibiotic therapy
- Observation for complications of sepsis: disseminated intravascular coagulation, renal failure, heart failure, GI ulcers, hepatic abnormalities

Chapter 21

Malignant Cerebral Edema

Scope of the Problem
Cerebral edema results from an increase in the fluid content of the brain. Metastasis to the brain is the prime source of cerebral edema. Primary tumors that metastasize to the brain most often are

- lung,
- breast,
- melanoma, and
- renal carcinoma.

Physiological Alterations
Cerebral edema can result from

- direct injury to vascular endothelium,
- dysplastic vascular structures within tumor,
- biochemical alteration of capillary permeability, and
- a less stable blood-brain barrier.

When cerebral edema exceeds the limits of compensatory mechanisms, brain herniation can occur.

Clinical Manifestations
Signs and symptoms of cerebral edema

- Headache
- Nausea and vomiting
- Weakness
- Personality changes
- Somnolence
- Impaired cognition

- Seizures
- Gait disorder
- Visual disturbance
- Language disturbance
- Hemiparesis
- Sensory loss (unilateral)
- Papilledema
- Ataxia
- Aphasia

Assessment and Diagnostic Measures

Neurological examination, computed tomographic (CT) scan, and magnetic resonance imaging (MRI) are common diagnostic studies. MRI is best for visualizing edema. Stereotactic needle biopsy may be required to obtain tissue for definitive diagnosis.

Treatment

Aggressive therapy is necessary to sustain or restore optimal neurological function.

Steroids, Anticonvulsants, and Osmotherapy

The single most important adjunctive treatment to combat the effects of cerebral edema is the use of glucocorticoids.

- High doses of dexamethasone (30 to 60 mg) is given in four to six divided doses to rapidly reduce the rate of fluid formation.
- The dose is tapered once neurological symptoms are controlled and reduced.

Patients who have seizures are placed on anticonvulsant therapy. Control of seizures avoids sudden increases in intracranial pressure.

Mannitol osmotherapy can be used to produce profound reduction of cerebral edema on a temporary basis.

PART IV

Surgery
Surgical decompression or debulking of the tumor is effective for reducing intracranial pressure and preventing further edema.

Radiation Therapy
Many unifocal brain tumors are potentially curable with radiation therapy. Tolerance of normal brain tissue is the dose-limiting factor. Radiation causes an acute increase in brain edema, characterized by headache, nausea, vomiting, and worsened neurological condition temporarily.

Interstitial brachytherapy with seeds (^{120}iodine or ^{192}iridium) to boost the field is occasionally used.

Chemotherapy
Several agents are effective but are limited by their inability to cross the blood–brain barrier and by toxicity.

Chapter 22

Malignant Peritoneal Effusion

Scope of the Problem

Malignant peritoneal effusion (ascites) occurs when fluid accumulates in the peritoneal space. Gynecological tumors account for about 75% of malignant ascites in women. Peritoneal effusion is usually a sign of advanced disease.

Tumors associated with peritoneal effusion

- Ovarian
- Uterine
- Cervical
- Pancreatic
- Gastric
- Colorectal

Physiological Alterations

Causes of peritoneal effusion

- Tumor seeding in the peritoneum
- Excess intraperitoneal fluid production
- Tumor as the cause of increased capillary leakage of proteins and fluids into the peritoneum
- Hypoalbuminemia and low serum protein

Clinical Manifestations

Several liters of fluid can accumulate in the peritoneal space.

Symptoms usually start to develop after 1 L of accumulation, such as the following:

- Weight gain (can be as much as 50 pounds)
- Distended abdomen
- Early satiety and indigestion

- Swollen ankles
- Fatigue
- Shortness of breath
- Fluid wave
- Shifting dullness
- Bulging flanks
- Everted umbilicus

Assessment
Typical measures for assessment and diagnosis

- Physical examination
- Abdominal x-ray
- Ultrasound
- Abdominal CT
- Paracentesis to obtain fluid for cytology

Treatment
The only effective treatment for peritoneal effusion is control of the primary tumor causing the effusion. If the patient is asymptomatic, the approach is to wait and see. If the patient is symptomatic, definitive therapy will be started and involves the following:

Paracentesis
- The goal is to remove accumulated fluid.
- Fluid can reaccumulate rapidly if tumor control is not possible.
- Risk of protein depletion and electrolyte abnormalities results from fluid removal.
- There is a risk of infection from an invasive procedure.

Obliteration of the Intraperitoneal Space
- The goal is to prevent fluid accumulation.
- Instillation of chemotherapeutic agents (e.g., cisplatin, bleomycin) administered into the peritoneum with a large-bore catheter, usually a Tenkhoff for long-term placement.

- Use of a Groshong catheter to drain ascites is another alternative.

Peritoneovenous Shunting
- Shunts are used to recirculate ascitic fluid to the intravascular space.
- This procedure is usually reserved for patients for whom other treatment options have failed.
- Complications of shunting include the following:
  - Clotting (most frequent problem)
  - Disseminated intravascular coagulation
  - Pulmonary embolism
  - Infection
  - Shunt malfunction

Chapter 23

Malignant Pleural Effusion

Scope of the Problem

Malignant pleural effusion occurs when a malignant process prevents reabsorption and fluid accumulates in the intrapleural space. A pleural effusion may be the initial symptom of a cancer, or the effusion may signal advanced disease. Malignant pleural effusion typically recurs unless the underlying disease is controlled or cured.

Approximately 50% of all cancer patients will develop a pleural effusion during the course of their disease. Most patients (90%) will have an effusion of more than 500 mL, and one-third will have bilateral effusions. Pleural effusion occurs most often with the following tumors (in order of incidence):

- Lung
- Breast
- Adenocarcinoma, primary unknown
- Leukemia, lymphoma
- Reproductive tract
- Gastrointestinal tract
- Genitourinary tract
- Primary unknown

Physiological Alterations

The causes of malignant pleural effusion typically involve the following:

- Implantation of cancer cells on the pleural surface leads to increased capillary permeability.
- Obstruction of lymphatic channels by tumor can prevent fluid resorption.

- Tumor obstruction of pulmonary veins can lead to increased capillary hydrostatic pressure.
- Necrotic tumor cells shed into pleural space can increase the colloid osmotic pressure.
- Thoracic duct perforation can produce chylous pleural effusion.

Clinical Manifestations

The extent of alteration of respiratory function depends on the amount and rate of fluid accumulation. Typical indicators

- Dyspnea
- Orthopnea
- Dry, nonproductive cough
- Chest pain, chest heaviness
- Labored breathing
- Tachypnea
- Dullness to percussion
- Restricted chest wall expansion
- Impaired transmission of breath sounds

Assessment

The methods typically used to assess and diagnose the occurrence of pleural effusion include any combinations of the following:

- Chest x-ray
- Examination of pleural fluid
- CT
- Ultrasound
- Thoracoscopy with direct pleural biopsy

Grossly bloody effusion is the strongest indicator of malignancy. Laboratory analysis of the pleural fluid is the only way to definitively diagnose the effusion.

Treatment

General guidelines for treatment indicate that small asymptomatic effusions be left alone, that responsive tumor types be treated, and, most importantly, that the patient's overall prognosis be the critical factor in determining the aggressiveness of management.

Control of the underlying cancer is the only way to definitively treat pleural effusion.

- Treatment is based on the specific tumor type and the previous cancer therapies.
- If the tumor type causing the effusion is chemoresponsive, systemic chemotherapy is initiated.
- However, if the tumor is questionably responsive, a trial of systemic chemotherapy is initiated to evaluate its effectiveness.
- If the tumor is chemoresistant or refractory to systemic treatment, pleurodesis is performed.

Thoracentesis
- Thoracentesis provides short-term relief of symptoms caused by a pleural effusion.
- Pleural fluid is removed by needle aspiration or via an implanted port through the chest wall.
- Potential complications of the thoracentesis include pneumothorax, pain, hypotension, or pulmonary edema.

Thoracostomy Tube
- Another measure to provide short-term relief of symptoms by periodically removing accumulated fluid

Obliteration or Sclerosis of the Pleural Space
- This involves instilling chemical agents that cause the visceral and parietal pleura to permanently adhere.
- The sclerosing agents most commonly used are bleomycin, doxycycline, and sterilized talc.

Other Methods

- Biological agents such as interferon
- Placement of indwelling, small-bore drainage catheters
- Pleural stripping is 90% effective in selected cases.
- A pleuroperitoneal shunt can also be inserted to divert pleural fluid into the subcutaneous tissue via a valved pump.
- External beam radiation can be used if the underlying tumor is responsive to radiotherapy. Pulmonary fibrosis is a potential complication of the radiation.

PART IV

Chapter 24

Nutritional Disturbances

Scope of the Problem

Undernutrition is the most common nutritional problem in the patient with cancer. Forty percent to 80% of patients with cancer develop some degree of malnutrition during their illness. Overnutrition is most common in breast cancer; 40% to 70% of women with breast cancer who are receiving adjuvant chemotherapy are reported to gain weight.

Cancer-associated cachexia can be differentiated into primary and secondary types.

- Primary cachexia results from tumor-produced metabolic abnormalities or host responses.
- Secondary cachexia results from mechanical effects of the tumor or treatment.

Risk Factors

Risk factors for malnutrition among cancer patients

- Age, body image, a history of eating disorders, social support, educational level, and the presence of comorbid diseases.
- Twenty percent to 30% of patients with non-Hodgkin's lymphoma have significant weight loss.
- Cancer of the aerodigestive and gastrointestinal tracts are at risk for undernutrition from mechanical obstruction and physiological dysfunction.
- Surgery alters function, which may reduce oral intake.

- Ileus may occur, reducing the ability to take in adequate nutrition.
- Malabsorption of fat, inadequate caloric intake, vitamin B12 deficiency, anemia, and fluid–electrolyte imbalance may occur with resections of the bowel.
- Radiation effects include anorexia, diarrhea, bleeding, nausea, vomiting, weight loss, mucositis, esophagitis, gastritis, xerostomia, and taste changes.
- Fatigue and appetite changes are common.
- Delayed effects of radiation include intestinal strictures, fibrosis or obstruction, fistulas, and hepatic or pulmonary fibrosis.
- Chemotherapy can cause stimulation of the chemotherapy receptor zone, causing nausea, vomiting, and anorexia.
- Biotherapy can cause anorexia, malaise, mucositis, nausea, and vomiting. Fatigue and flu-like symptoms are common.

Physiological Alterations

Cancer, the patient's response, and the cancer treatment alter the normal physiology.

Cancer-Induced Changes

- Loss of appetite may be related to the production of cytokines (e.g., tumor necrosis factor) by the cancer.
- Altered taste and smell sensors may affect appetite.
- Electrolyte imbalance may occur, producing altered appetite and taste changes.
- Excessive energy requirements of tumors cause greater energy expenditures for individuals.
- Cancer can cause abnormalities in carbohydrate, protein, and lipid metabolism.
- Cancers of the aerodigestive structures can cause decreased food and nutrient intake asso-

ciated with difficulty chewing or swallowing, obstruction, dysmotility, fistulas, tumor infiltration, or protein-losing enteropathy.

Treatment-Induced Changes

- Biotherapeutics such as tumor necrosis factor, interferon, and interleukins may affect appetite.
- Surgical anesthesia, chemotherapy, and radiation produce indirect effects on appetite, causing anorexia, nausea, vomiting, diarrhea, constipation, and food aversions.
- Nutritional needs increase as the body responds to repair damage induced by therapeutic interventions.

Clinical Manifestations

The most common clinical manifestation identified with cancer is cancer cachexia, which is characterized by anorexia, weight loss, skeletal muscle wasting, and reduced function. Other symptoms include early satiety, edema, anemia, reduced attention span, organ dysfunction, metabolic abnormalities, and susceptibility to other diseases.

Assessment

- Medical history would include the duration and type of malignancy as well as any complications such as infections or draining lesions. The type of treatment, such as radiation, chemotherapy, antibiotics, or surgical intervention, are noted.
- Laboratory assessment includes a complete blood count, a comprehensive metabolic panel, creatinine clearance and creatinine height index, and a delayed hypersensitivity response.
- Anthropometrics assesses the weight, size, and proportions of the body. Serial weight measurement is the single most important indicator of nutritional status. Skin-fold thickness and

body-part circumferences to assess fat and muscle compartments are usually measured by a dietician.

- Other physical parameters of nutrition include condition of hair, skin, teeth, mouth, gums, and throat and general performance status.

- Dietary history includes a 24-hour recall of foods eaten as well as a diet diary and calorie count. Past or current diet modifications, any special diets or vitamin supplements, or food allergies or intolerances are noted.

Treatment

Verbal counseling and education are effective in assisting patients in choosing appropriate calorie-dense foods to manage symptoms that interfere with oral intake. Certain medications may help to boost the appetite. For example, megestrol acetate has been found to improve appetite, cause weight gain, control nausea, and improve quality of life among individuals with cancer. Dosages range from 160 to 800 mg/day.

Approaches to Problems That Interfere with Normal Nutrition

- General
  - Drink plenty of fluids while avoiding empty-calorie foods, such as soda. Eating high caloric nutritious foods early in the day is recommended because generally energy is highest then. Mealtime should be pleasant, and the food should be attractive, with adequate flavoring.

- Dysphagia
  - Eat soft or liquid foods, "blenderize" solid foods, and moisten foods with cream, gravies, or oils. Eating bland foods that are smooth in texture and tepid will minimize pain.

- Nausea and vomiting
  - Avoid acidic foods or overly sweet, greasy, or high-fat foods. Eat salty, dry foods such as

toast or crackers. Eat small, frequent meals slowly. Eat frozen juice sticks and drink clear, cool beverages for fluid. Wear loose clothing and take antinausea, antiemetic, and tranquilizing medications as prescribed.

- Early satiety
  - Eat five or six small meals per day that are high in calories and low in fat. Drink nutritious liquids, such as juice, milk, or milkshakes either 30 minutes before or after meals. Chew foods slowly, and avoid greasy foods.

- Anorexia
  - Eat small, frequent meals that are varied. Try new recipes or foods that are highly nutritious. Take medications with high-calorie foods or nutritional supplements. Stimulate the appetite with light exercise or drink a small glass of wine or fruit juice before meals.

- Dumping syndrome
  - Eat small meals containing foods that are low in concentrated carbohydrate but high in protein. Avoid liquids with meals.

- Constipation
  - Drink at least 2 L of fluid daily, and consume high-fiber foods. Increase exercise and take previously successful bowel stimulants.

- Diarrhea
  - Drink at least 2 L of fluid daily, but avoid milk or milk products unless they are treated with lactase enzyme. Electrolyte replacement fluids may be necessary if diarrhea persists. Avoid foods that are high in fiber or those that are high in fat, spicy, and gas-forming. Eat electrolyte-rich foods.

- Dyspepsia
  - Avoid foods that are high in fat, spicy, or citrus. Elevate the upper trunk after meals and use antacids liberally.
- Stomatitis
  - Eat soft or liquid foods, preferably cold or frozen to numb the pain. Avoid irritating foods or liquids that are rough, acidic, or hot. Cleanse the oral cavity frequently (every 2 to 3 hours) with warm saline irrigants.
- Taste changes
  - Substitute poultry, fish, eggs, or cheese for red meat if there is an aversion to red meat. Serve meats chilled rather than hot. Try marinating foods to increase flavor. Use high-protein liquid supplements if meat is not tolerated. Try extra spices, onion, or garlic to improve the flavor of food. Rinse the mouth with carbonated water or a lemon wedge before meals to clear the palate. Try using plastic rather than metal utensils if food tastes like metal.
- Xerostomia
  - Moisten foods with gravies or sauces and swallow liquid with each bite of food. Blenderize or process foods to make them easier to eat. Soak foods in coffee, tea, milk, or a similar beverage. Use a humidifier or steam kettle in the room where food is eaten. Artificial saliva may also be helpful.

Enteral Nutrition (Tube Feeding)

Enteral feeding is indicated if oral intake cannot prevent weight loss or if a person's physical condition prevents oral intake. A functioning gastrointestinal (GI) tract is required.

For tumors of the upper aerodigestive tract, placing the feeding tube directly into the small intestine may be indicated. For more permanent feeding, a surgically placed esophagostomy, gastrostomy, or jejunostomy tube may be indicated.

Formulas may be prepared from regular food or may be commercially prepared.

Side effects from enteral feedings lessen over time. Problems and solutions with enteral feedings include the following:

- *Diarrhea:* Give formula at room temperature; use a lactose-free formula. Antidiarrheal medication is indicated. Fluid and electrolyte disturbances may occur.

- *Hyperglycemia* may occur during the initial stages of feeding and may continue in individuals with diabetes.

- *Regurgitation:* Check tube placement; withhold feedings if residual is more than 100 to 200 cc; keep in Fowler's position; use a small bore tube; place the tube distally and consider drugs to increase motility.

- *Nausea:* Check tube placement; reduce the rate; change the formula and consider blenderizing table foods, which tend to be easier to digest; review other potential sources on nausea, such as infection or medications.

- *Distention:* Use a low-fat or hydrolyzed formula; encourage activity; review other potential sources of distention, such as obstruction, constipation, or organomegaly.

- *Dehydration:* Increase water intake to ensure adequate amounts and to control diarrhea.

- *Tube obstruction:* Use room-temperature feedings; irrigate with water. Use a pump with high-density formulas or small-bore tubes; use liquid medicines rather than crushing pills, whenever possible.

Total Parenteral Nutrition

Total parenteral nutrition (TPN) is indicated for individuals without a functioning gastrointestinal tract, such as those with severe enteritis following radiation, high-output fistulas, malabsorption secondary to aggressive cancer therapy or obstructed bowel but otherwise acceptable quality of life.

Complications and solutions of parenteral feedings include the following:

- *Pneumohemothorax:* Put the patient in the Trendelenburg position for line placement; check the x-ray postprocedure.
- *Embolism:* Follow the flushing regimen; avoid use of small-diameter syringes when flushing; avoid exposure to free air.
- *Metabolic abnormalities:* Monitor levels of glucose, ammonia, phosphate, liver enzymes, magnesium, and potassium hemoglobin/hematocrit.
- *Hyperglycemia* occurs in 15% of patients receiving TPN; it occurs when the infusion is too rapid or there are increased insulin demands on the individual. Monitor with fractional urine tests or finger sticks every 6 hours. Symptoms include dry mouth, flushed skin, thirst, malaise, polyuria, nausea, or vomiting. Hyperglycemia is treated by adding insulin to the TPN solution.
- *Hypoglycemia* occurs when too much insulin is administered or when TPN infusion is interrupted or discontinued shortly after insulin is given. Symptoms include headache, drowsiness, dizziness, tachycardia, and tremor.
- *Essential fatty-acid deficiency* occurs as a result of prolonged reduction of fat intake. Administer lipid emulsion to individuals who receive TPN for longer than 14 days without dietary fat intake.
  - Do not use emulsion if color or texture is inconsistent.
  - Nothing can be added to a lipid infusion.
  - Infuse in the same line as the TPN solution, using a Y-connector.
  - Do not use a filter.

PART IV

- Maximum rate of infusion is 1 cc/min for first 30 minutes. If there are no untoward reactions, increase to the rate of 500 cc over 4 to 12 hours.

- Observe for allergic reactions, dyspnea, cyanosis, nausea, vomiting, headache, flushing, fever, chills, pain in the chest or back, irritation at the infusion site, and diaphoresis. Discontinue infusion if any allergic reaction occurs.

- *Infection:* Perform careful site care and evaluation; monitor temperature, glucose levels, glucosuria. Offending organisms are usually skin microorganisms, such as the bacteria *Staphylococcus, Klebsiella,* and *Corynebacterium* species and the fungi *Candida* species. Clinical signs of sepsis include fever, hypotension, tachycardia, and tachypnea.

  - If there is a temperature spike, peripheral blood and blood drawn from catheter are cultured for the presence of bacteria and fungi.

  - The catheter is removed if cultures are positive. A new catheter is not inserted until all blood cultures show negative results.

  - Appropriate antibiotics and antifungal agents are given as indicated.

Chapter 25

Assessment of Cancer Pain

Scope of the Problem

Pain is one of the most prevalent symptoms faced by patients with cancer. Pain is more prevalent in those patients with advanced disease (e.g., lung and breast cancer) and those being treated in hospice or specialty units. Pancreatic and primary bone cancer exhibit high prevalence rates of pain across all stages of disease.

Pain has been defined as an unpleasant sensory and emotional experience associated with tissue damage. Chronic pain and acute pain are different. Pain is a multidimensional phenomenon that contributes to the patient's perception of and response to pain.

PART IV

Obstacles to Successful Pain Management

Obstacles to pain management can be attributed to health care professionals, patients and family, and the health care system. These obstacles include the following:

- Lack of understanding about pain
- Expectation that pain should be present
- Relief of pain not viewed as a goal of treatment
- Inadequate or nonexistent assessment
- Undertreatment with analgesics
- Inadequate knowledge of analgesics and other drugs
- Fears of addiction, sedation, and respiratory depression
- Inadequate knowledge of other interventions for pain

- Perceptual differences between patients and health care providers
- Legal impediments

Principles of Assessment and Management

Nurses play an important role in the assessment and management of pain. The nurse's role includes

- describing pain,
- identifying aggravating and relieving factors,
- determining the meaning of pain and determining its cause,
- determining individuals' definitions of optimal pain relief,
- deriving nursing diagnoses,
- assisting in selecting interventions, and
- evaluating the efficacy of interventions.

In addition to the nurse's role, other principles of assessment and management that are necessary for successful nursing management of cancer pain include

- an interdisciplinary approach in delivery of pain-management services,
- a well-defined scope of nursing practice,
- thorough assessment and documentation,
- incorporation of guidelines and standards into clinical practice,
- evaluation of outcomes, and
- approaches to managing pain in special populations.

Assessment and Documentation

There are six dimensions to the cancer pain experience that need to be assessed:

1. *Physiological dimension*
   - Onset

- Type of pain (e.g., somatic, visceral, neuropathic, breakthrough)
- Duration (acute pain: self-limiting; chronic pain: lasting 3 months or longer)
- Associated factors
- Syndrome
- Anatomy and physiology

2. *Sensory dimension*
   - Location of pain
   - Intensity (e.g., mild, moderate, severe)
   - Quality (e.g., burning, stabbing, throbbing)
   - Pattern (e.g., intermittent, constant, transient)

3. *Affective dimension*
   - Distress
   - Anxiety
   - Depression
   - Mental state
   - Perception of suffering
   - Irritability/agitation
   - Pain relief

4. *Cognitive dimension*
   - Meaning of pain
   - Thought processes
   - Coping strategies
   - Knowledge, attitudes, beliefs
   - Previous treatments
   - Influencing factors (positive and negative)
   - Level of cognition and/or impairment

5. *Behavioral dimension*
   - Activities of daily living
   - Behaviors (pain-related, preventive, controlling)
   - Use of medications
   - Sleep and rest patterns

PART IV

- Fatigue and other symptoms
6. *Sociocultural dimension*
   - Ethnocultural background
   - Family and social life
   - Work and home responsibilities
   - Environment
   - Familial attitudes, beliefs, and behaviors
   - Personal attitudes, beliefs, and behaviors
   - Communication with others
   - Interpersonal relationships

Standardized pain assessment tools and documentation procedures facilitate management of pain. Children, elderly patients, individuals with a history of substance abuse, individuals from diverse cultural backgrounds, and terminally ill patients require special consideration in pain assessment and management.

Chapter 26

Management of Cancer Pain

New developments have led to advances in the use of pharmacotherapy, nonpharmacological approaches, and invasive interventional techniques in the management of cancer pain.

Interventions and techniques for managing cancer pain can be categorized into three major approaches:

- Treat the underlying pathology to control, reduce, or eradicate the tumor.
- Change the perception or sensation of pain using pharmacological and interventional techniques.
- Diminish the emotional or reactive component to alter the central processing of pain.

PART IV

Treatment of Underlying Pathology

The three major treatment modalities (chemotherapy, radiation therapy, and surgery) are effective in the control and palliation of cancer pain.

1. Chemotherapy to palliate symptoms
   - Hormonal therapy can provide relief of painful bony metastases from breast and prostate cancers.
2. Radiation therapy provides fast pain relief in patients with
   - bone, brain, and hepatic metastases;
   - epidural cord compression; and
   - nerve root infiltration.
3. Surgery is a palliative measure to
   - resolve oncologic emergencies,
   - reduce tumor burden,

- provide direct access to tumor (e.g., implants of infusion pumps or radiation seeds),
- prevent and repair fractures from metastatic disease, and
- interrupt the pain pathway.

Change in Perception/Sensation of Pain

Pharmacological Therapy

Nonopioids

Nonopioids are nonsteroidal antiinflammatory drugs (NSAIDs) used alone or with an opioid for

- mild to moderate pain,
- metastatic bone pain,
- pain from compression of tendons, muscles, pleura, and peritoneum, and
- visceral pain.

Commonly used nonopioids

- Acetaminophen
- Acetylsalicylic acid
- Choline magnesium trisalicylate
- Diclofenac
- Diflunisal
- Ibuprofen
- Indomethacin
- Ketorolac
- Naproxen

Major toxicities of NSAIDs

- Gastrointestinal (GI) disorders: nausea, vomiting, epigastric pain, ulcers, bleeding, diarrhea, constipation
- Renal dysfunction
- Sodium and water retention
- Skin rashes
- Headaches

Steroids

Steroids can be effective for problems such as bone metastases, compression from solid tumors, lymphedema, and brachial and lumbosacral plexopathies. It is generally recommended that steroids be reserved for those patients with advanced disease or for short-term use.

Opioid Agonists

Opioid agonists are very useful for cancer pain. Various patient-related factors contribute to the selection of a specific opioid (i.e., pain intensity, age, concomitant medical illnesses, and characteristics of drug). Specific drugs and considerations

- Morphine (most frequently used opioid for moderate to severe cancer pain)
- Fentanyl
- Hydromorphone (useful alternative to morphine for the elderly)
- Methadone (choice opioid for patients allergic to morphine; not recommended for the elderly because of its long plasma half-life).
- Oxycodone

Common side effects of opioid analgesics
- Sedation, drowsiness, mental clouding, lethargy
- Respiratory depression (treat with naloxone)
- Nausea and vomiting
- Constipation (a significant problem with opioid therapy; the use of laxative preparations is generally necessary).

Routes of opioid administration
- Oral route (sublingual, transmucosal)
  - Convenient and safe
  - Inexpensive
  - Should be used for as long as possible
  - Sublingual route can be used intermittently

PART IV

for short-term management of breakthrough pain

- Transmucosal route is now possible with oral transmucosal fentanyl citrate.

- Transdermal route (fentanyl is only opioid available via this route)
- Rectal route
- Parenteral (intramuscular, subcutaneous, intravenous) route
  - Occasional intramuscular or subcutaneous injection for immediate pain relief if no peripheral or central venous access
  - Consider continuous infusion if analgesic needed every 2 hours or less
  - Continuous intravenous infusions provide steady blood levels of opioid.
  - Continuous subcutaneous infusions are an acceptable alternative when intravenous access is limited, patients are unable to take oral medications, or oral medications do not provide control. Morphine, hydromorphone, and methadone are the most common opioids used for continuous subcutaneous infusions.
  - Patient-controlled analgesia (PCA) allows patients to self-administer analgesics from a special infusion pump. PCA is used with intravenous and subcutaneous routes and avoids highs and lows of (PRN) administration. Indications for appropriate use for PCA are when the patient wants self-control, when the oral route is not available, and for breakthrough pain.
- Intraspinal (epidural, intrathecal) opioid administration: Criteria for intraspinal opioids include the following:
  - Unacceptable toxicities from systemic opioids
  - Neuroablative or anesthetic procedures unsuccessful or not indicated

- Good home and family support
- Life expectancy of more than 3 months

Adjuvant Analgesics

Adjuvant analgesics are those medications that enhance the action of pain-modulating systems. The most common agents

- *Antidepressants* are used for neuropathic pain (e.g., continuous burning) caused by tumor infiltration of nerves:
  - Amitriptyline
  - Doxepin
  - Nortriptyline
  - Desipramine
- *Anticonvulsants* are used for lancinating and stabbing neuropathic pain. Commonly used drugs:
  - Gabapentin
  - Phenytoin
  - Clonazepam
  - Carbamazepine
  - Valproic acid
- *Psychostimulants* are useful for counteracting the sedation from opioid analgesics:
  - Amphetamines
  - Methylphenidate

Bisphosphonates

Bisphosphonates (e.g., clodronate, pamidronate) relieve bone pain and improve outcomes for patients with metatstatic bone involvement.

Nerve Blocks and Neuroablative Procedures
- Temporary or nondestructive nerve blocks are used for treatment of intractable pain, but relief is short-term.
- Neurolytic or destructive nerve blocks provide prolonged pain relief and are useful for treating pain that is well-defined or localized.

PART IV

- Destructive neurosurgical procedures (e.g., peripheral neurectomy, cordotomy, rhizotomy) are used when standard pharmacological and nonpharmacologcial strategies are no longer effective.

Diminishing the Emotional and Reactive Components of Pain

Interventions included in this approach do not affect pathology or alter sensation or perception of pain, but decrease patients' emotional responses to pain so they can deal with pain more effectively. These nonpharmacological techniques are adjuvant to standard pharmacological therapy and are within the scope of nursing practice.

Cutaneous Stimulation

These methods are thought to help relieve pain by physiologically altering the transmission of stimuli:

- Heat
- Cold
- Massage
- Transcutaneous electrical nerve stimulation (TENS)

Immobilization and Mobilization

Complete or partial immobilization of the body or parts of the body may relieve pain. On the other hand, mild exercise may help decrease pain.

Distraction

This method involves diverting one's attention away from sensations or feelings related to pain. Distraction strategies

- Conversation
- Visualization and imagery
- Breathing exercises
- Counting, reading, watching television
- Speaking to others

- Music therapy
- Humor

Relaxation and Guided Imagery
The two most common methods for relaxation training

- Progressive muscle relaxation (tensing and re-laxing 16 muscle groups)
- Self-relaxation (passive, quiet, and still use of autogenic phrases)

Guided imagery is the visualization of pleasant places or things and is used with relaxation techniques.

Education and Information
Accurate and appropriate pain education for patients and families is essential for pain management. The Agency for Health Care Policy and Research guidelines suggest appropriate content for pain education.

PART IV

Part V

Oncologic Emergencies

Chapter 27

Cardiac Tamponade

Scope of the Problem
Cardiac tamponade is a life-threatening oncologic emergency that results from an excess accumulation of fluid in the pericardial sac (pericardial effusion). This fluid causes an increase in pressure around the heart and a decrease in blood flow to the heart.

Etiology and Risk Factors
The most common cause of cardiac tamponade is malignancies. Tumors associated with the development of pericardial effusions include lung (40%), breast (23%), lymphoma (11%), and leukemia (5%). Cardiac tamponade can also result from constriction of the pericardium by tumor or postradiation pericarditis.

Physiological Alterations
The amount of fluid surrounding the heart can range from 50 mL to greater than 1 L. As excess fluid accumulates, it compresses the right ventricle and it cannot fill. This results in a decrease in blood leaving that chamber. Therefore, the amount of blood entering and leaving the left side of the heart is decreased. The severity of cardiac tamponade is based on the rate of fluid accumulation and the amount of fluid that accumulates.

Clinical Manifestations
The signs and symptoms of cardiac tamponade are variable and depend on the rate and amount of pericardial fluid accumulation and the individual's baseline cardiac function (Table 27.1).

Table 27.1 **Pathological Responses of Cardiac Tamponade and Clinical Presentations**

Pathology	Signs and Symptoms
Decreased cardiac output	Increased resting heart rate decreases cardiac output.
	Peripheral vasoconstriction shunts blood to vital organs.
	Decreased renal output with decreased renal perfusion
	Narrowing pulse pressure as arteries constrict to maintain perfusion
	Paradoxical pulse occurs because the left ventricle receives less blood and cardiac output is reduced.
	Anxiety, restlessness, and confusion occur because of cerebral anoxia.
	Symptoms of shock occur as the heart decompensates.
Compression of heart and structures	Dysphagia
	Cough
	Retrosternal chest pain
Venous congestion due to decreased ventricular output	Peripheral edema
	Jugular venous distention
Distention and filling of the pericardial sac	Weak heart sounds
	Chest fullness and discomfort

Assessment

Diagnostic tests include the following:

- Echocardiography is the most sensitive and precise method for the diagnosis of cardiac tamponade.
- Radiograph may reveal an enlarged heart, mediastinal widening, dilated cardiac silhouette, cardiomegaly, and pleural effusions.
- Computerized tomography (CT) may indicate the presence of a cardiac tamponade, pericar-

dial thickening, and the presence of a pleural effusion.

- Magnetic resonance imaging reveals a more defined view of the myocardium, compared with CT.
- Pulmonary artery catheterization reveals hemodynamic changes within the heart.
- Serum laboratory tests, including hematocrit and arterial blood gas, may reveal bleeding or respiratory alkalosis with an increase in pH.
- Pericardial fluid evaluation is usually done under ultrasound guidance and is done to determine the etiology of the effusion.

Treatment

The goals of treatment include enhancing cardiac function, pericardial fluid removal, prevention of reaccumulation, and minimizing complications. Treatment approaches include the following:

- Pericardiocentesis is performed to remove the fluid from the pericardial sac. A catheter may be left in place to facilitate drainage of the effusion.
- Pericardiocentesis with sclerosing is done to prevent reaccumulation of fluid. Instillation of sclerosing agents such as bleomycin, doxycycline, or radioisotopes creates an inflammatory response of the pericardium.
- Pericardiotomy, the insertion of a balloon catheter into the pericardial sac, temporarily prevents reaccumulation of fluid.
- Pleuropericardial window involves removal of a piece of the pericardium, which allows fluid to drain from the pericardial sac if the effusion recurs.
- Pericardiectomy involves resection of the pericardium to facilitate drainage of fluid into the pleural space.

Nursing Measures

Nursing measures are designed to address the following patient-related problems:

- Decreased cardiac output related to decreased ventricular filling
  - Assess for signs and symptoms of decreased cardiac output, such as decreased blood pressure, increased heart rate, decreased level of consciousness, and shortness of breath.
  - Monitor blood pressure, heart rate, respiratory rate, central venous pressure, and pulmonary artery pressures.
  - Assess cardiac rhythm and ECG.
  - Administer aggressive fluid therapy.
  - Administer supplemental oxygen.
- Altered tissue perfusion related to decreased cardiac output
  - Assess for cool skin, altered mental status, and increased capillary refill time.
  - Monitor arterial blood gas (ABG) results for acid-base imbalance.
  - Administer supplemental oxygen.
- Impaired gas exchange related to pericardial effusions
  - Assess for mental status changes, tachypnea, tachycardia, dyspnea, and orthopnea.
  - Monitor ABG results and administer supplemental oxygen.
  - Monitor vital signs hourly and prn.
  - Provide measures to minimize anxiety.
- Potential for infection related to procedure and antineoplastic therapy
  - Assess for signs and symptoms of infection, including fever, tachycardia, tachypnea, increased WBCs, redness or discharge from catheter sites, and positive blood culture results.

PART V

- Maintain aseptic or sterile technique with indwelling catheter care.
- Administer antibiotic therapy as prescribed.
- Perform sterile dressing changes according to institutional policy and procedure.
- Anxiety related to procedures, symptoms and critical nature of illness, and possible lack of information
  - Encourage the patient to verbalize feelings.
  - Explain all procedures and clarify misconceptions.
  - Allow time for exchange of information.
  - Administer anxiolytics.
  - Explain all procedures and rationale for symptoms.
  - Assess individual understanding of information.
  - Provide written education information regarding symptoms and procedures.

Chapter 28

Disseminated Intravascular Coagulation

Scope of the Problem

Disseminated intravascular coagulation (DIC) represents an inappropriate and exaggerated overstimulation of normal coagulation, in which both thrombosis and hemorrhage may occur simultaneously. DIC occurs in approximately 10% of persons with cancer and is nearly always secondary to an underlying disease process.

Etiology and Risk Factors

DIC in the cancer population is always secondary to the malignancy or to an underlying condition such as infection. Associated conditions in cancer are summarized as follows:

- Infection and sepsis are the most common causes of DIC and can be bacterial, fungal, and viral in origin. Sepsis from gram-negative bacteria is the most frequent cause of DIC.
- Intravascular hemorrhage related to blood transfusion reactions or multiple transfusions of whole blood can lead to renal failure, shock, DIC, and severe bleeding.
- Acute leukemia and adenocarcinomas, such as cancers of the lung, breast, stomach, and prostate, are commonly associated with DIC.
- Liver disease that results in hepatic failure disrupts the normal balance of coagulation and increases the risk of DIC.
- Prosthetic devices, such as a peritoneovenous shunt that shunts ascitic fluid into the systemic circulation, can trigger DIC.

PART V

Physiological Alterations

Once the coagulation system is activated, thrombin, the central proteolytic enzyme of blood coagulation, is produced.

Steps critical to the process of DIC:

- Fibrinogen is consumed by thrombin-induced clotting and plasmin-induced fibrinolysis.
- Decreased macrophage-clearing function limits removal of activated clotting factors.
- Rapid coagulation exceeds the ability of liver to clear fibrin split products (FSPs), and excess FSPs inhibit clotting.
- Consumable factors I, II, V, and VIII are depleted by microvascular clotting.

Acute DIC in a hemodynamically unstable patient is characterized by microvascular thrombosis and bleeding from multiple sites occurring simultaneously.

Clinical Manifestations

DIC is often a fatal process, as it frequently goes unrecognized until severe hemorrhage occurs. Bleeding is the most obvious sign of a hemorrhagic disorder and can occur from any orifice.

Early Signs and Symptoms
- Anxiety, restlessness
- Tachycardia, tachypnea, and headache
- Conjunctival hemorrhage and periorbital petechiae
- Oozing blood and bleeding gums

Late Signs and Symptoms
- Change in mentation
- Frank hematuria
- Joint pain
- Hemoptysis, tarry stool, or melena

Major Complications
- Bleeding with the potential for hemorrhage, resulting in hypoxia, acidosis, hypotension, proteinuria, and altered fluid balance
- Thrombus formation

Assessment
DIC is defined by the presence of two or more of the following abnormalities:

- Prothrombin time increased by 3 or more seconds over control time
- Activated partial thromboplastin time increased by 5 or more seconds over control time
- Thrombin time prolonged by 3 or more seconds over control time
- Fibrinogen less than 150 mg/dL
- Fibrin split products equal to or greater than 40 µg/mL
- Decreased platelet count

Treatment
Treatment of the underlying malignancy is vital because the tumor is the underlying stimulus; all other measures are only supportive.

Supportive Measures
- Give platelets and fresh-frozen plasma to replace consumed blood components.
- Give fresh-frozen plasma and antithrombin III concentrate to neutralize excess thrombin and slow the DIC process.
- Although considered controversial therapy, heparin (7.5 U/kg/hr) may be given as a continuous infusion or as a low dose subcutaneously to stop the intravascular clotting process.
- Heparin use is contraindicated if there is any sign of intracranial bleeding (e.g., headache), open wounds, or recent surgery.

PART V

- Heparin infusion is stopped immediately if the person complains of headache or displays signs of frank bleeding.
- ε-Aminocaproic acid is controversial, but may be given if the preceding measures fail to maintain platelet and fibrinogen levels.
- ε-Aminocaproic acid is not used in most cases because inhibition of the fibrinolytic system can lead to widespread fibrin deposition in microcirculation.

Effective control of DIC is measured by normal coagulation screen and platelet count.

General Nursing Measures
- Monitoring vital signs, urine output, and blood loss.
- Administer medications to suppress symptoms (e.g., cough, vomiting) that increase intracranial pressure.
- Initiate bleeding precautions.
- Monitor for signs of cardiogenic shock: hypovolemia, hypoxia, hypotension, and oliguria.

Chapter 29

Septic Shock

Scope of the Problem

Septic shock is a systemic blood infection characterized by hypotension, hypoxemia, and organ dysfunction that persists despite aggressive fluid challenge. Septic shock develops in approximately 27% to 46% of patients with gram-negative bacteremia, resulting in inadequate tissue perfusion and circulatory collapse. The mortality rate is 75% for cancer patients who develop septic shock.

Etiology and Risk Factors

The incidence of sepsis is increasing as a result of numerous invasive procedures and aggressive antineoplastic therapies that ultimately cause multiple immune defects.

Risk factors for septic shock

- Malignancy (leukemia/lymphoma)
- Immunosuppression
- Granulocytopenia is the single most important risk factor for sepsis in individuals with cancer. A granulocyte count of less than 500/mm^3 is associated with the greatest risk of septic shock.
- Upper or lower respiratory infection
- Mucositis
- Urinary tract infection
- Invasive procedures

Physiological Alterations

The pathogenesis of septic shock is complex and not completely understood. As the invading organism interacts with the immune system, factors from the damaged organism and host immune system factors enter the bloodstream and damage the lining of the blood vessels. The most important bacterial factor is endotoxin, and the most important immune response factor is tumor necrosis factor, which damage the lining of blood vessels and lead to shock.

As septic shock progresses, fibrinolysis, coagulopathies, and possibly DIC may occur. Venous pooling, decreased venous return, and maldistribution of blood volume are responsible for the classic symptoms of hypotension observed in septic shock.

Clinical Manifestations

The classic symptoms of septic shock include fever, shaking chills, hypotension, tachycardia, tachypnea, and mental status changes.

Organ dysfunction in septic shock generally presents with early and late symptoms, which are listed in Table 29.1.

Table 29.1 Organ Dysfunction in Septic Shock	
System	**Manifestations**
Central nervous system	Severe sepsis presents as apprehension, confusion, disorientation, and agitation, and progresses to obtundation and coma in septic shock.
Cardiovascular	Sinus tachycardia and increased blood pressure in severe sepsis lead to dysrhythmias and hypotension with a normal or high cardiac output in septic shock. Cardiac collapse can occur.
Pulmonary	Tachypnea and hypoxia with respiratory and metabolic acidosis give way to shortness of breath, pulmonary edema, and acute respiratory distress syndrome.
Renal	A decreased urine output and increased osmolality in severe sepsis develop into oliguria, anuria, elevation of BUN and creatinine, and acute renal failure.

Hematological	Leukopenia, thrombocytopenia and prolonged PT/PTT, a decreased fibrinogen, and elevation in fibrin degradation products lead to a worsening in the symptoms of DIC in septic shock.
Metabolic and electrolyte	Temperature elevation, lactic acidosis, and hyperglycemia lead to severe electrolyte imbalance, hyperglycemia, and worsening of lactic acidosis.

Assessment

The key to preventing progression from infection to septic shock is early recognition and intervention.

- Blood cultures are done to identify microorganisms and are repeated every 24 hours if septic shock persists.
- Echocardiograms, CT scans, a ventilation/perfusion scan, and chest radiographs are done to evaluate organ function and determine the infectious source.
- Frequent monitoring of the complete blood count, electrolytes, lactic acid, arterial blood gases, and coagulation profiles provide information about the severity of septic shock.

Treatment

Major therapeutic goals in septic shock management

- Hemodynamic support involves providing adequate circulating volume to raise the blood pressure and enhance cardiac performance and normalization of oxidative metabolism.
- Treatment of the infection involves prompt and appropriate initiation of antibiotics.
- Oxygenation of tissues is critical as interstitial and alveolar edema worsen, and ventilation/perfusion mismatch increases oxygen demand.

PART V

Chapter 30

....

Spinal Cord Compression

Scope of the Problem

Spinal cord compression (SCC) is a malignant process that causes disruption in neurologic function when a tumor and its destructive effects on the vertebral column compress neural tissue and its blood supply. Approximately 5% to 10% of cancer patients develop SCC. Over 95% of SCC cases are caused by tumor that has metastasized to the vertebral column. Partial or complete paralysis may occur if SCC is not recognized or treated early. The majority of patients are paralyzed at the time of diagnosis and fewer than 25% will regain their ability to ambulate.

The incidence may be increasing due to improved treatments and prolonged survival. The incidence is highest among patients with cancers that metastasize to bone, especially the vertebrae, such as breast, lung, sarcoma, and prostate cancers.

Physiological Alterations

SCC occurs by direct extension of the tumor into the epidural space, vertebral collapse and displacement of bone into the epidural space, or by direct extension through the intervertebral foramina.

SCC can arise from either primary tumors within the spinal cord or as a result of metastatic disease. Primary tumors of the spine that arise within the cord itself are called intramedullary, and those that develop within the dural layers are called extramedullary–intradural.

Epidural metastasis is the most common type of metastasis to the spine. The vertebral column is the most common site for skeletal metastasis. The thoracic spine is the most frequent site of epidural compression.

The site of cord compression is related to the primary cancer, for example:

- Cervical compression is most often caused by metastatic breast cancer.
- Thoracic compression is most often caused by metastatic lung, breast, and prostate cancer.
- Lumbosacral compression is most often caused by metastatic gastrointestinal (GI) cancers.

Clinical Manifestations

Physical Assessment

The manifestations of SCC depend on the level of the lesion and compression. The initial symptom is back pain accompanied or followed by motor weakness and decreased sensation. Weakness progresses to motor and sensory loss, loss of proprioception, vibratory sense, and bowel and bladder dysfunction. Assessment of SCC should consider the following:

- Back pain, the presenting symptom in over 95% of patients with SCC, can be localized or radiate from one location to another.
- Cervical and lumbosacral compression usually presents with unilateral radicular pain.
- Thoracic compression is usually associated with bilateral radicular pain.
- Back pain from cord compression may be elicited with movement, the valsalva maneuver, cough, and straight leg raising or neck flexion.
- Back pain from cord compression differs from degenerative disease in that lying supine does not alleviate the pain.

PART V

- Assessment of back pain includes percussing the vertebrae and having the patient perform leg raising or neck flexion, a description of the nature and character of the pain, its intensity, and its alleviating and aggravating factors.
- Numbness or paresthesias are early symptoms of cord compression.
- Sensory loss is accompanied by loss of proprioception, position sense, vibration, temperature sense, and deep pressure.
- Disruption of lower motor neuron function is a late sign of SCC and includes sphincter problems that result in bowel and bladder incontinence or retention.

Diagnostic Evaluation
- Plain films and bone scans will demonstrate vertebral body collapse, pedicle erosion, and osteolytic or osteoblastic lesions in more that 83% of cases of epidural metastasis.
- For plain films to demonstrate osteolytic osseous destruction, greater than 50% of bone must be affected.
- Magnetic resonance imaging (MRI) is the preferred tool for the diagnosis of SCC. If an MRI is not available, a myelogram with CT scan is comparable.

Treatment
The single most important prognostic indicator with SCC is neurological status before initiation of therapy; the less extensive the injury to cord, the greater the potential for recovery. Effective treatment generally involves one or more of the following: steroids, radiation, surgical interventions, and chemotherapy.

Steroids
- Steroids relieve pain and improve neurologic function by reducing spinal cord edema.

- Dosing for steroids is a bolus of dexamethasone 10 mg intravenously, followed by 4 mg every 6 hours.

Radiation
- The usual dose range is 2000 to 4000 cGy given in 5 to 20 fractions.
- The side effects of radiation are related to myelosuppression, skin reactions, and nausea and or heart burn, depending on the location of the port.

Surgical Interventions
- Surgical decompression and laminectomy or vertebral body resection can promptly relieve SCC.
- Surgical intervention is intended to completely resect the tumor and reconstruct the spine. The spine may be stabilized with bone grafting or fusion.
- The goal of surgical intervention is to relieve pain and provide spinal stability that allows full ambulation and neurological recovery.
- Complications of surgery include infection, cerebrospinal fluid leakage, progression of neurological deficits, instrumentation or stabilization failure, and hemorrhage.

Chemotherapy and Other Systemic Therapies
- Chemotherapy may be used as adjunctive therapy to radiation.
- Hormonal manipulation treatments for breast cancer and prostate cancer may be beneficial.
- Bisphosphonates delay the onset and reduce the frequency of skeletal-related episodes such as pathological fracture, bone pain, and SCC.

Nursing Measures
- Pain management is achieved with pharmacological and nonpharmacological measures.

PART V

- Protection of the patient from sensory, motor, or neurological injury
- Rehabilitation needs depend on the pretreatment status of the patient. If pretreatment neurological status is poor, the patient will not likely regain function.
- Extensive rehabilitation can aid in maximizing recovery or providing adaptive measures.

Chapter 31

Superior Vena Cava Syndrome

Scope of the Problem

Superior vena cava syndrome (SVCS) refers to signs and symptoms that occur when blood flow through the superior vena cava is compromised. Venous congestion and restricted cardiac output occur proximal to the obstruction. Respiratory distress and/or cerebral edema due to SVCS constitute an oncologic emergency.

SVCS occurs in only 3% to 4% of individuals with cancer. While the majority of patients with SVCS have cancer, 15% to 22% of cases are caused by thrombus formation and compression of the superior vena cava by a benign process.

Etiology and Risk Factors

The most common types of cancer associated with SVCS are lung cancer, lymphoma, and metastatic breast cancer. SVCS occurs in 3% to 10% of all individuals with lung cancer. Individuals with right lung cancer are more likely to develop SVCS than are those with left lung cancer, because the superior vena cava is nearer to the right lung.

Increased incidence of catheter-related thrombosis occurs when the catheter tip is in the upper half of the vena cava and the catheter is placed on the left side. The left brachiocephalic vein forms a more marked angle with the vena cava, and the wall of the vena cava may be injured with catheter insertion.

Physiological Alterations

Obstruction of the superior vena cava is caused by external compression by primary or metastatic

PART V

193

cancer, direct invasion by tumor, or thrombus formation within the vessel. Any obstructive process that reduces venous blood return to the heart from the upper body will increase venous congestion and decrease cardiac output.

Development of SVCS depends on the following:

- Degree and location of the obstruction
- Aggressiveness of the tumor
- Competency of collateral circulation

If untreated, SVCS can lead to thrombosis, cerebral edema, pulmonary complications, and death.

Clinical Manifestations

Gradual, slow progression of obstruction causes slow onset of symptoms due to the development of collateral circulation that compensates for the obstruction.

Early Signs and Symptoms

- Shortness of breath
- Tachypnea
- Nonproductive cough
- Neck vein distention
- Swelling of face, neck, arms, and hands
- Periorbital edema
- Mild headache, anxiety, and lightheadedness, especially on exertion

Late Signs and Symptoms

- Stridor
- Respiratory distress
- Facial flushing
- Anxiety
- Dysphagia with or without hemoptysis
- Tachycardia
- Decreased or absent peripheral pulses
- Congestive heart failure, decreased blood pressure, and cyanosis

- Severe headache, visual disturbances, mental status changes, seizures, and papilledema

Assessment

Physical Examination

- Physical examination often reveals the classic clinical findings of SVCS, which are neck vein distention, chest wall vein distention, edema of the face and upper extremities, and periorbital edema. Bending over, stooping, or lying flat may aggravate symptoms.
- Physical assessment may also reveal plethora, facial flushing, cyanosis, dizziness, and tachypnea.
- Individuals with catheter-related thrombosis may experience shoulder or retrosternal pain exacerbated by injection into the catheter.

Diagnostic Studies

- Diagnostic tests include chest x-ray, computerized tomography, fiberoscopy, lymph node biopsy, mediastinoscopy, and thoracotomy. Mediastinoscopy and thoracotomy are performed only when other procedures are inconclusive and cancer is suspected.
- A chest x-ray may reveal a mediastinal mass or adenopathy with or without mediastinal widening. Pleural effusion due to venous hypertension and thoracic lymphatic obstruction also may be found.
- Histopathologic diagnosis via biopsy or cytology will establish the diagnosis of cancer in approximately 70% of cases.

Treatment

Treatment of SVCS is based on the cause of the obstruction, severity of symptoms, prognosis, patient preferences, and goals of treatment.

Thrombolysis

SVCS in catheter-related thrombosis is treated with infusion of a thrombolytic agent such as

PART V

streptokinase, urokinase, or tissue plasmino-
gen activator and heparin. Patients are monitored for bleeding and central nervous system
effects.

Chemotherapy
Multidrug chemotherapy is effective in the treatment of SVCS caused by small cell lung cancer
and non-Hodgkin's lymphoma. Upper extremity
intravenous access may not be optimal due to
compression of the venous system. Patients are
monitored for infection due to myelosuppression,
nausea and vomiting, stomatitis, esophagitis, and
alopecia.

Radiation Therapy
Radiation therapy for SVCS is often administered
for 2 to 3 days as high-dose fractions of 4 Gy and
as daily fractions of 1.8 to 2.0 Gy until the total
prescribed dose is complete (30 to 50 Gy in 3 to 5
weeks). Steroids are sometimes given to reduce
edema.

Early side effects include esophagitis, cough, nausea, skin reactions, and fatigue. Late effects of radiation to the mediastinum include pneumonitis,
pulmonary fibrosis, esophageal ulceration or
stenosis, cardiac changes, spinal cord myelopathy,
and brachial plexopathy.

Stent Placement
Intravascular placement of self-expanding stents
is done to relieve SVC obstruction. Ninety-two
percent of patients experience improvement of
symptoms within 12 hours of stent placement.
Resolution of peripheral edema occurs within
1 to 7 days. Recurrent SVC obstruction is observed
in up to 45% of cases, possibly due to malignant
invasion through the stented area. Complications
of stent placement include groin hematoma or
infection and femoral site deep vein thrombosis.

Nursing Measures

The goals of nursing care

- Ongoing assessment of status
- Maintenance of adequate cardiopulmonary function
- Maximization of oxygenation and perfusion
- Provision of comfort measures to relieve dyspnea and anxiety

Chapter 32

Syndrome of Inappropriate Antidiuretic Hormone

Scope of the Problem
Syndrome of inappropriate antidiuretic hormone (SIADH) is described as tumor production of antidiuretic hormone (ADH) or its biological active form, arginine vasopressin (AVP), resulting in hyponatremia, hyperosmolality of the urine, and high urinary sodium.

SIADH is a rare emergency, occurring in only 1% to 2% of cancer patients. It is primarily associated with small cell lung cancer.

Etiology and Risk Factors
SIADH is caused by the ectopic production of vasopressin by malignant cells. Nonmalignant causes of SIADH include infectious diseases (pneumonia, tuberculosis, and empyema), pain, nausea, emotional stress, drugs (vincristine, vinblastine, cyclophosphamide, morphine), and general anesthesia, all of which increase AVP production.

Physiological Alterations
Normally, the body maintains fluid volume and concentration within a very narrow range regulated by AVP on the kidney. When AVP is present, the collecting duct is permeable to water, resulting in water reabsorption and concentrated urine. Suppression of AVP leads to urine dilution.

Cancer cells have the ability to store and release AVP, and excess AVP leads to water intoxication. Water intoxication leads to a decrease in plasma osmolality, dilutional hyponatremia, increased urinary excretion of sodium, and further hyponatremia. Intracellular edema occurs as the plasma water follows an osmotic gradient. Cerebral edema occurs and leads to a disruption of neural function and death.

Clinical Manifestations

Water intoxication accounts for the symptomatology of SIADH.

- Moderate hyponatremia (serum sodium level of 115 to 129 mEq/L)
  - Nausea, thirst, headache, weakness, anorexia, fatigue, and muscle cramps
  - Symptoms progress to changes in mental status, such as confusion, lethargy, combativeness, or psychotic behavior.
- Severe hyponatremia (100 to 110 mEq/L)
  - Seizures, coma, and death

Assessment

The diagnosis of SIADH is most often made concurrently with the discovery of the malignancy.

Criteria for the diagnosis of SIADH

- Serum osmolality of < 275 mOsm/kg; serum sodium < 130 mEq/L
- Urine osmolality where urinary sodium is > 25 mEq/L and euvolemia
- Decreased levels of BUN, uric acid, creatinine, and albumin
- Absence of edema and normal renal, adrenal, and thyroid function

PART V

Treatment

Successful treatment of the underlying malignancy is the only potential cure for SIADH. The severity of the hyponatremia and water intoxication determine the treatment of SIADH.

Mild Hyponatremia

- Fluid restriction to 800 to 1000 mL/day is the initial treatment of mild hyponatremia and may be the only therapy necessary.

Severe Hyponatremia

- Fluid restriction to 500 mL in 24 hours and administration of hypertonic 3% saline solution and furosemide intravenously are necessary.
- Serum sodium and electrolytes are checked every 1 to 3 hours.
- Once fluid/electrolyte balance and neurological status are stabilized, begin chemotherapy.

Chronic Mild to Moderate Hyponatremia

- SIADH that persists despite initial therapy may be treated with demeclocycline (900 to 1200 mg/day). Demeclocycline inhibits the action of ADH and induces reversible diabetes insipidus. Absorption is affected by foods high in calcium, and the drug should be taken on an empty stomach.

Nursing Measures

- Administration of chemotherapy
- Management of side effects
- Patient and family education regarding self-care measures, including recognition of the early signs and symptoms of hyponatremia

Chapter 33

Tumor Lysis Syndrome

Scope of the Problem

Tumor lysis syndrome (TLS) is a metabolic complication of effective cancer therapy that occurs when large numbers of tumor cells are destroyed rapidly. Tumor cell destruction causes high levels of intracellular components—primarily potassium, phosphorus, and uric acid, to be released into the bloodstream.

Metabolic abnormalities can develop alone or in combination.

- Hyperuricemia can lead to renal tubular obstruction/acute renal failure.
- Hyperkalemia can lead to lethal cardiac arrhythmias.
- Hyperphosphatemia may result in acute renal failure.
- Hypocalcemia (related to hyperphosphatemia) can cause muscle cramps, cardiac arrhythmias, and tetany.

Etiology and Risk Factors

The most frequent cause of TLS is the administration of systemic chemotherapy that causes rapid cell lysis, and necrosis of a tumor mass can induce this syndrome.

Risk factors

- Tumor characteristics
  - Large tumor burden
  - High growth fraction
  - Lymphoma, leukemia (These cells are highly chemosensitive and lyse rapidly during induction therapy, and immature lymphoblasts

PART V

contain abnormally high levels of phosphorus.)

- Patient characteristics
  - High white cell count
  - Lymphadenopathy
  - Splenomegaly
  - Preexisting renal impairment
  - Elevated uric acid, phosphate, and potassium
- Cancer treatment characteristics
  - Effective chemotherapy
  - High-dose chemotherapy
  - High-log cell kill

Physiological Alterations

When tumor cells lyse, there is a release of a large amount of phosphorus into the blood, causing a proportional decrease in serum calcium, resulting in hypocalcemia. Acute renal failure is secondary to hyperuricemia and hyperphosphatemia.

Uric acid nephropathy occurs because uric acid crystals form in the collective ducts of the kidneys and ureter, leading to obstructive uropathy with decreased glomerular filtration, increased hydrostatic pressure, obstructed urine flow, and acute renal failure.

Renal insufficiency exacerbates hyperkalemia and hypocalcemia. Hyperkalemia depresses cardiac function, resulting in bradycardia, heart block, and cardiac arrest.

Clinical Manifestations

The four major clinical manifestations of TLS are hyperuricemia, hyperkalemia, hyperphosphatemia, and hypocalcemia. The severity of these metabolic alterations is related to tumor burden and renal dysfunction.

Early Manifestations
- Fatigue/lethargy
- Nausea, vomiting, anorexia
- Diarrhea
- Flank pain, muscle weakness, and cramps

Late Manifestations
- Ascending flaccid paralysis
- Oliguria, anuria, and hematuria
- Edema
- Azotemia
- Laryngospasm, tetany, and convulsions
- Bradycardia, hypotension, cardiac arrest, and death

Assessment
Initially, a complete history and physical is performed and risk factors for TLS are identified. Patients at high risk of developing TLS may require hospitalization for their treatment.

Specific laboratory parameters evaluated prior to, during, and after treatment include the following:

- Serum potassium, phosphorus, calcium, uric acid, blood urea nitrogen, creatinine, LDH, complete blood count, and platelet count
- Monitoring of renal function and cardiac function throughout treatment

Treatment
The primary goal of TLS management is prevention. Preventive measures reduce the risk of severe electrolyte imbalances. Following are the four key elements of TLS prevention and intervention.

Aggressive Hydration and Diuresis
- Patients are hydrated with at least 3 L/m^2/day to ensure a urinary output of 100 to 200 cc/hour.

- Diuretics are used to maintain urinary flow and prevent renal tubular damage while promoting excretion of potassium, phosphate, and uric acid and inhibiting calcium reabsorption.
- Vigorous hydration begins 24 to 48 hours prior to treatment and continues for several days posttreatment.

Allopurinol
- Allopurinol inhibits the enzyme xanthine oxidase and prevents the formation of uric acid, which prevents uric acid nephropathy.
- Allopurinol 300 to 500 mg orally or intravenously is given several days before, during, and after cytotoxic therapy.

Urinary Alkalinization
- Add 50 to 100 mEq of sodium bicarbonate to each liter of intravenous hydration and/or administer acetazolamide 250 to 500 mg intravenously daily.
- Alkalinization increases the solubility of uric acid.

Early Identification and Correction of Electrolyte Imbalances
- Frequent laboratory assessment of electrolytes and renal function
- Assessment of the signs and symptoms of TLS

Part VI

The Care of Individuals with Cancer

Chapter 34

AIDS-Related Malignancies

Approximately 40% of persons living with AIDS will experience an AIDS-related malignancy. The three most common malignancies in AIDS that are discussed in this chapter are Kaposi's sarcoma (KS), non-Hodgkin's lymphoma (NHL), and cervical cancer.

KAPOSI'S SARCOMA

Incidence
Since the AIDS pandemic, more than 24,000 cases of AIDS-associated KS have been reported to the Centers for Disease Control. KS has been reported in 40% of homosexual/bisexual men, 11% of heterosexual men, and 2% of women. The incidence is declining, and, to date, KS is seen in 14% of all cases of AIDS.

Etiology
Several risk factors are implicated in the development of KS:

- Sexually transmitted cofactor spread via receptive anal sex
- Immunosuppression
- Genetic predisposition may exist
- Herpes virus type 8 (HHV-8)

Pathophysiology
HIV disease causes the infected mononuclear cell to synthesize a whole range of inflammatory cytokines and angiogenic factors. These create a climate in which KS cells grow, leading to widespread disease.

Clinical Manifestations
- Lesions first appear on the upper body as pink or red oval bruises or macules that become dark blue and spread to the oral cavity and lower body.
- Lesions may be painless, nonpruritic, and palpable.
- Lymphatic involvement can result in severe edema.
- Gastrointestinal involvement can result in protein-losing enteropathy.
- Pulmonary involvement leads to respiratory distress.

Assessment
Suspicious lesions are biopsied before a diagnosis of KS is made. Several factors are associated with a poorer prognosis:
- CD4 cell count < 200/mm^3
- History of AIDS prior to development of KS
- History of systemic "B" symptoms (i.e., fever, nightsweats, weight loss)

Treatment
The pace of the disease is variable and specific treatments are begun as necessary (Table 34.1).

Table 34.1 Cancer Treatments Based on Extent of Disease

Extent of Disease	Treatment
Few, small lesions	No treatment; watch and wait
Few lesions, cosmetically or psychologically unacceptable	Cosmetic makeup; surgical excision; local treatments (cryotherapy, laser therapy, hCG, local injections of vinblastine, interferon, or vincristine)
Extensive mucocutaneous KS with or without asymptomatic visceral disease	Radiation therapy; interferon plus antiretrovirals

PART VI

continued

Rapid progression of disease; symptomatic visceral disease, pulmonary KS; lymphedema	Single or multiple chemotherapy agents: doxorubicin, bleomycin, vincristine (ABV); liposomal daunomycin or doxorubicin; paclitaxel

Supportive Care

Patient education and psychosocial support are of utmost importance. Body image disturbances are frequent, and patients may become extremely depressed. The obstructive, compressive, and progressive nature of the tumor will dictate the range of care.

NON-HODGKIN'S LYMPHOMA

Incidence

Lymphoma is the second most common cancer in HIV (following KS). The incidence of NHL among persons with HIV/AIDS is much higher than in the general population. It is frequently the initial AIDS-defining diagnosis. NHL is the cause of death in 16% to 20% of HIV-infected persons.

Etiology

NHL occurs in all populations of persons with AIDS, regardless of the manner in which HIV was contracted. There is a slightly higher incidence in

- men who have sex with men,
- individuals with a history of injecting drugs,
- white men,
- increasing age, and
- the immunosuppressed.

Pathophysiology

HIV infection induces B-cell stimulation, proliferation, and activation. The majority of AIDS-related NHL begin as B-lymphocyte malignant neoplasms. The most common sites of AIDS-related NHL are the

- brain (43% of all AIDS-related NHL),
- heart, and
- anorectal area.

Clinical Manifestations

The majority of patients (74%) present with weight loss, nightsweats, and unexplained fever. Fatigue and lymphadenopathy are common. NHL of the brain is associated with hemaparesis, mental status changes, headache, or seizures.

Assessment

Biopsy specimens, resected tissue, or cytologic examination of tissue fluid determines diagnosis and classification. The diagnostic work-up includes the following:

- History, physical examination
- Laboratory tests
- Chest x-ray
- Bone marrow biopsy
- Lumbar puncture
- Computed tomographic (CT) scans of the chest, abdomen, and pelvis
- MRI of the brain

Factors associated with decreased survival

- Elevated serum lactate dehydrogenase
- Karnofsky scores less than 50%
- Age over 35 years
- CD4+ T-cell count less than 100/mm^3
- History of an AIDS-defining illness prior to lymphoma

PART VI

Treatment

The treatment for AIDS-related NHL is difficult because of the presence of immunosuppression, poor bone marrow reserve, and increased risk for opportunistic infections.

- CNS lymphoma: The treatment of choice is radiation therapy.
- Low-dose chemotherapy regimens are the treatment of choice for the majority of patients.
- Administration of colony-stimulating factors is effective in reducing associated bacterial and fungal infections.

Supportive Care

Care is the same as for those with non–AIDS-related NHL. Care of patients with CNS lymphoma involves the following:

- Monitor focal findings, motor incoordination, and cognitive deficits.
- Establish a safe environment in the acute and home settings.
- Provide emotional support to patient and family.
- Plans may be needed for transfer to a skilled nursing care facility.
- If the patient is legally incompetent, a legal guardian must be appointed.

CERVICAL CANCER

Incidence

Women represent the fastest rising population at risk for HIV/AIDS in the United States. The true incidence of invasive cervical cancer is unknown.

Etiology

There are multiple risk factors for the development of cervical intraepithelial neoplasia (CIN) and cervical cancer in HIV-infected women

- Early age at intercourse
- Multiple sex partners
- Sex with men who have sex with multiple partners

- Injecting drug users
- Cigarette smoking
- Dietary deficiencies
- Immunosuppression
- Low socioeconomic status
- Lack of access to health care
- History of sexually transmitted disease
- Exposure to diethylstilbestrol in utero

Pathophysiology
The early stage of the disease involves the microinvasion of the lesion into the basement membrane of the cervix. CIN and cancer of the cervix progress from mild dysplasia (grade I) to moderate dysplasia (grade II), to severe dysplasia and carcinoma in situ (grade III).

Clinical Manifestations
There are no symptoms in the early stages of CIN. The most common symptoms of cervical cancer include the following:

- Postcoital bleeding
- Metorrhagia and vaginal discharge
- Abdominal, pelvic, back, or leg pain
- Anorexia, weight loss
- Edema of the legs
- Anemia

Assessment
The Pap smear is the primary screening tool. Other diagnostic measures include endocervical curettage, conization, colposcopy, and biopsy.

Treatment
Definitive therapy for CIN II or III includes the use of cryotherapy, carbon dioxide, laser therapy, cone biopsy or loop excision, and simple hysterectomy. Optimal therapy for invasive cervical cancer is

not yet known but may include the combination strategies of surgery, radiation, and chemotherapy.

Supportive Care

Continued assessment and follow-up are necessary. Patients should be counseled about safe sex and potential decisions regarding pregnancy and childbirth.

Chapter 35

Bladder Cancer

Incidence
Bladder cancer is the second most common genitourinary cancer after prostate cancer. It occurs four times more often in men than in women and is more common in whites than in blacks. The average age at diagnosis is 65.

Etiology

Risk Factors
- Cigarette smoking
- Occupational exposure to industrial chemicals
- Exposure to the parasite *Schistosoma* (rare in the United States)
- Exposure to other carcinogenic agents

Pathophysiology
Approximately 90% to 95% of bladder cancers are transitional cell carcinomas that arise in the epithelial layer of the bladder. The growth rate of bladder tumors depends on histological type, tumor grade, and depth of bladder wall invasion. The 5-year survival rate ranges from 94% for those with localized disease to 6% for those with distant metastasis.

PART VI

Clinical Manifestations
- Hematuria (may be gross or microscopic)
- Dysuria
- Urinary frequency, urgency, and burning
- Decrease in urinary stream

- Flank, rectal, back, or suprapubic pain (usually with advanced disease)

Assessment

There are no early signs of bladder cancer on physical examination unless it is an invasive mass revealed by rectal examination. Diagnostic tests establish the presence of a bladder mass. The most useful diagnostic tests include the following:

- Urine cytology, flow cytometry
- Excretory urogram
- Cystoscopy
- Computerized tomography (CT) scan
- Magnetic resonance imaging (MRI)
- Tumor markers (*p53,* blood group antigens, epidermal growth factor) may be useful in predicting response to treatment and recurrence.

Classification and Staging

The TNM system and the Jewett-Marshall system are two staging systems used for bladder cancer.

Treatment

The treatment selection depends on stage and grade of tumor. The treatment for carcinoma in situ (CIS); superficial, low-grade tumors; and invasive tumors is summarized as follows.

Carcinoma In Situ

- Transurethral resection
- Intravesical therapy with thiotepa, bacillus Calmette-Guérin (BCG), mitomycin C, or doxorubicin
- Radical cystectomy with urinary diversion (for high-grade, poorly differentiated CIS)

Superficial, Low-Grade Tumors

More than 75% of patients present with superficial tumors.

Treatment options

- Transurethral resection (TUR) and fulguration with or without intravesical chemotherapy, laser therapy, or cystectomy
- Intravesical therapy with chemotherapeutic and immunotherapeutic agents (e.g., thiotepa, BCG, mitomycin C, or doxorubicin). Interferons, bropirimine, keyhole-limpet hemocyanin, and photodynamic therapy are being evaluated.
- Laser therapy
- Partial cystectomy, which preserves bladder and male erectile function

Invasive Tumors

Invasive bladder cancer represents muscle invasion and requires aggressive therapy.

Treatment options

- Radical cystectomy with urinary diversion with or without pelvic lymph node dissection. There are several types of urinary diversion, including the incontinent ileal conduit and the continent urinary reservoir.
- Definitive radiotherapy
- Combination chemotherapy either before or after surgery and radiotherapy. The combination of methotrexate, vincristine, doxorubicin, and cisplatin (MVAC) has shown good outcomes. Other agents being evaluated include gemcitabine, taxanes, ifosfamide, 5-fluorouracil, trimetrexate, and piritrexim.

Supportive Care

Preoperative nursing care involves selection of the stoma site and teaching the patient self-catheterization. Postoperative care depends on the method used to create a urinary diversion or bladder.

Postsurgical Sexuality

A radical cystectomy with urinary diversion can affect many aspects of sexual functioning such as:

- Impotency in men
- Narrowing and dryness of the vagina in women
- Change in body image due to the stoma and appliance

Insertion of a penile prosthesis may help erectile impotence. Ample lubrication and using different positions during intercourse may decrease pain and discomfort in women.

Urinary Diversion with Ileal Conduit
The viability (color) of the stoma needs to be assessed regularly. The continuous outflow of urine requires the individual to wear an appliance at all times. Good skin care is essential. Teaching the patient continuing care of a conduit and periodic reevaluation of the stoma, peristomal skin, and function of the conduit can avoid many complications.

Continent Urinary Reservoir
The continent urinary reservoir produces much mucus and needs regular irrigation in the early postoperative period; mucus decreases over time. No appliance is necessary. Patient teaching focuses on self-catheterization of the pouch, stoma care, and care of the catheter if the reservoir is attached to the skin. If the reservoir is attached to the urethra, the patient is instructed on voiding technique, schedule of voiding, Kegel exercises, and self-catheterization in the event of urinary retention due to mucus.

Chapter 36

Bone and Soft Tissue Sarcomas

Incidence
The American Cancer Society estimates 2900 new cases of bone cancer and 8700 new cases of soft tissue cancer in 2001. The estimated number of deaths from bone cancer is 1400, and 4400 from soft tissue tumors.

Etiology
The cause of bone and soft tissue cancers is not known.

Established risk factors
- High-dose radiation
- Chemicals, such as vinyl chloride gas, arsenic, and dioxin (Agent Orange) have been associated with soft tissue sarcomas.
- Family history is implicated in both bone and soft tissue sarcomas.
- Paget's disease is a risk factor, primarily for bone tumors.
- Skeletal maldevelopment and abnormal skeletal growth patterns are associated with bone sarcomas.
- Genetic predisposition may be a risk factor for certain sarcomas.

Pathophysiology
Primary malignant bone and soft tissue tumors are derived from cells of the mesoderm and the ectoderm and include the following tumors.

Osteosarcoma (Osteogenic Sarcoma)
- Arises from the osteoblasts
- Most common osseous malignant bone tumor

PART VI

- Greatest incidence between 10 and 25 years of age
- Incidence twice as high in men as in women
- Incidence increased in adults with Paget's disease
- Most common sites: distal femur, proximal tibia, and proximal humerus
- Metastasis primarily to the lungs
- Five-year survival rates: 10% to 20%
- Adjuvant chemotherapy after surgery increases disease-free survival.

Chondrosarcoma
- Arises from chondroblasts
- Accounts for approximately 14% of malignant bone tumors
- Incidence greatest among males age 30 to 60
- Associated with syndromes of skeletal maldevelopment
- Most frequent sites: pelvic bone, long bones, scapula, and ribs
- Most remain localized and slow growing
- Metastasis occurs to the lungs.

Fibrosarcoma
- Arises from fibroblasts
- Accounts for fewer than 7% of primary malignant bone tumors
- Rare in children
- No gender predominance
- Paget's disease and therapeutic radiation may be predisposing factors.
- Femur and tibia are the most common sites of occurrence.
- Metastasis occurs to the lungs.
- Surgery is the treatment of choice.
- Fibrosarcomas are considered radioresistant.

Ewing's Sarcoma

- Arises from the bone marrow reticulum
- Accounts for 6% of all malignant bone tumors
- 80% are diagnosed in individuals between the ages of 5 and 15.
- Males are affected more than females.
- Commonly located in the pelvis and diaphyseal or metadiaphyseal regions of long bones
- Metastasis may be present in 20% of individuals at diagnosis.
- Fever, anemia, high erythrocyte sedimentation rates, and leukocytosis may be present at diagnosis.

Soft Tissue Sarcoma

- Common soft tissue sarcomas include malignant fibrous histiocytoma, liposarcoma, fibrosarcoma, synovial sarcoma, rhabdomyosarcoma, and leiomyosarcoma.
- Occur primarily in the extremities; some also occur in the head and neck or retroperitoneum.
- Nodal metastasis is common.
- Metastasis occurs to the lungs, usually within the first 2 years of treatment.

Metastatic Bone Tumors

- Primary tumors that metastasize to bone include lung, melanoma, gastric, breast, colon, prostate, pancreatic, kidney, testicular, and thyroid.
- More common sites of metastases include the spine, pelvis, and ribs.
- Tumors spread to bone from the primary tumor either by direct extension to adjacent bones, arterial embolization, or direct venous spread through the pelvic and vertebral veins (Batson's plexis).

PART VI

Clinical Manifestations

Bone and soft tissue sarcomas can present with either a painful area on the musculoskeletal system, pain at rest, or a soft tissue or bony mass that may not be painful.

Assessment

Patient and Family History

Evaluation of the location, onset, duration, and quality of pain is a major focus.

- Bone pain often has a gradual onset unless it presents as a pathological fracture. Pain may be radicular and is often constant and worse at night.
- Soft tissue sarcomas often are painless masses unless they are impinging on nerves, blood vessels, or viscera.
- Hemoptysis, chest pain, or cough is suggestive of pulmonary spread.
- Any family history of Paget's disease or neurofibromatosis should be noted.

Physical Examination

Inspection of the affected area may reveal a visible mass or swelling. Dilated surface veins may be evident. A firm, nontender, warm enlargement may be noted. Evaluation for adenopathy, hepatomegaly, and neurovascular function of the affected limb is done.

Diagnostic Studies

Three basic patterns of tumor destruction may be viewed radiographically and are described as follows:

1. The geographic pattern is characterized by a large, well-defined hole where the destroyed bone interfaces with the intact bone. This indicates that the tumor has a slow rate of growth.

2. A moth-eaten pattern indicates a moderately aggressive tumor characterized by multiple

holes that tend to coalesce. Severe cortical destruction is present.

3. A permeative pattern indicates an aggressive tumor with a tendency to infiltrate. It is characterized by multiple tiny holes in cortical bone.

Other radiological methods include bone scans, arteriography, computerized tomography, fluoroscopy, and magnetic resonance imaging.

Biopsy may be obtained by use of an open (incisional) or closed (needle) technique.

Classification and Staging

Classification of bone and soft tissue tumors is based on histological patterns, radiological features, and biological behavior of the tumor. The American Joint Committee on Cancer has recommended the *International Histological Classification of Tumors* for specific definitions of histological typing. The staging system for musculoskeletal sarcomas includes surgical grade, surgical site, and presence of metastases.

- Stage I includes low-grade lesions with low incidence of metastases.
- Stage II includes high-grade lesions with high incidence of metastases. "A" indicates an intra-compartmental lesion; "B" indicates an extra-compartmental lesion.
- Stage III includes any site or grade lesion with metastases.

Treatment

Goals of treatment of primary malignant bone and soft tissue cancer include eradication of the tumor, avoidance of amputation when possible, and preservation of maximum function. The primary lesion is managed by surgery, radiotherapy, chemotherapy, or a combination.

PART VI

Surgery

Surgical management of primary bone cancer is strongly influenced by the histopathology and anatomical site.

Contraindications for limb salvage

- Inability to attain adequate surgical margin
- Neurovascular bundle involved by tumor
- Pathological fractures
- Children younger than 10 years because of resultant limb length discrepancy

Radical Resection with Reconstruction

Radical resection with reconstruction uses metal and synthetic materials as well as bone autografts or allografts.

The three most common methods of reconstruction after resection

1. *Arthrodesis* or *fusion* results in a stiff joint; however, it is sturdy and permits activities such as running and jumping.
2. *Arthroplasty with metallic or allograft implant* allows maintenance of joint function. The implant, however, is an artificial joint and will not tolerate stress.
3. *Intercalary allograft* reconstruction involves placement of an allograft between two segments of bone that is secured with metal plates.

Complications include blood loss, anemia, pain, possible wound necrosis, pneumonia, pulmonary embolism, and deep vein thrombosis. Limb elevation, length of bed rest, and other restrictions depend on the extent of the resection.

Radical Resection without Reconstruction

Amputations are indicated for patients with large, invasive tumors of the extremities. Amputation of the lower extremity will generally require an immediate or a delayed-fitting prosthesis.

- *An immediate-fitting prosthesis* involves a rigid dressing and cast applied at the time of surgery. A socket on the distal end of the cast attaches to the prosthetic unit. Usually, the patient experiences better emotional adjustment with the immediate fitting. However, the wound cannot be visualized easily and the temporary prosthesis is heavy.

- *Delayed fitting* involves a temporary or intermediate prosthesis at 3 to 6 weeks. Ambulation with weight bearing is encouraged. Three months after surgery, the individual is fitted with a permanent prosthesis. Advantages are that the wound can be inspected for healing. Disadvantages are that edema delays shrinking and shaping of the stump, and attention must be given to prevention of contractures.

Phantom limb pain is experienced by 35% of patients following amputation. It is characterized by severe cramping, throbbing, or burning pain in various areas of the amputated limb. It occurs 1 to 4 weeks after surgery and may be triggered by fatigue, excitement, sickness, weather changes, and stress. Pain worsens over time for 5% to 10% of amputees.

Radiotherapy

The use of radiotherapy in the management of primary or metastatic malignant bone or soft tissue sarcoma depends on the radiosensitivity of the particular tumor type. With the exception of Ewing's and soft tissue sarcomas, radiotherapy is generally reserved for palliation.

Complications of treatment

- Tendon contractures
- Edema of the involved extremity distal to the site of irradiation
- Cessation of growth of the extremity
- Nonhealing fractures

PART VI

Chemotherapy and Immunotherapy

Chemotherapy is given preoperatively and post-operatively. The rationale for preoperative chemotherapy is to treat the micrometastasis, to decrease the primary tumor size, thereby increasing the likelihood of limb salvage surgery, and to assess the effectiveness of the chemotherapeutic agents.

Osteosarcoma has been treated with doxorubicin, high-dose cyclophosphamide or high-dose methotrexate with leucovorin rescue, with a significant increase in 5-year survival.

Ewing's sarcoma has been treated with ifosfamide and etoposide or actinomycin, doxorubicin, vincristine, and cyclophosphamide in conjunction with radiation therapy and surgery.

Supportive Care

Pain

Pain management approaches

- Nonsteroidal antiinflammatory agents progress to mild opiates such as codeine, and, eventually, opiates such as morphine or methadone.
- Combinations of various classes of agents, such as a nonsteroidal antiinflammatory agent and an opiate with or without other agents, are appropriate.
- Walking aids may be used to minimize weight bearing of the involved limb.
- Pamidronate intravenously on a monthly basis may be helpful to decrease pain, promote bone healing, and minimize metastatic spread to bone.

Limitations of Mobility

Assistive devices such as a sling, crutches, or a cane may be necessary to support the involved area and prevent fracture. A wheelchair may facilitate out-of-home activities and maintain the same activity levels.

Arrangement for a home aide to assist with housekeeping and other care needs may be appropriate. Consultation with family members and home care agencies may be appropriate, depending on the physical abilities and rehabilitation goals of the patient.

Chapter 37

......•••••••

Breast Cancer

Incidence

Breast cancer is the leading cause of death in women 40 to 44 years of age. Incidence in the United States is 1 in 8 women. More than 70% of breast cancers occur in women 50 years of age and older. There is a slight increase in incidence of breast cancer in women under age 55 and in black women. It is second only to lung cancer as the leading cause of cancer deaths in women. Mortality rates have begun to decline more in white women than in black women.

Etiology

Risk Factors

Despite the identification of various risk factors for breast cancer, specifically the genetic and familial factors, approximately 50% of women who develop breast cancer have no identifiable risk factors beyond being female and over the age of 50.

Primary Risk Factors

- Female gender
- Fifty years of age and older
- A native of North America or northern Europe
- A family history of breast cancer
- A personal history of breast cancer
- Breast cancer in two or more first-degree relatives
- Bilateral or premenopausal breast cancer in a first-degree relative
- Breast cancer susceptibility genes, which appear to be transmitted in an autosomal dominant manner

- Mutations of *BRCA1*, *BRCA2*, and the *p53* tumor-suppressor gene

Secondary Risk Factors
- Postmenopausal obesity
- Menarche before age 12; menopause after age 55
- First full-term pregnancy after age 35
- Use of oral contraceptives before age 20 and persisting for 6 or more years
- Ionizing radiation exposure to the chest before age 35
- Benign breast disease

Other Risk Factors
- Nulliparity
- Ingestion of more than two alcoholic drinks per day
- High-fat diet in adolescence

Prevention
- Chemoprevention is the use of a chemical agent such as tamoxifen to prevent breast cancer in women at high-risk.
- The STAR (Study of Tamoxifen and Raloxifene) trial is designd to examine the effects of breast cancer risk reduction and relative side effects using tamoxifen versus raloxifene.
- Exercise may possibly have a protective effect against breast cancer, but more research is needed.
- Prophylactic mastectomy may be appropriate for some women who are at high genetic risk and psychologically distraught over the possibility of having breast cancer.

Pathophysiology

Cellular Characteristics
A majority of primary breast cancers are adenocarcinomas located in the upper outer quadrant

PART VI

of the breast. The most common types of breast tumors include the following:

- *Infiltrating ductal carcinoma* presents as a prominent lump, with stony hardness on palpation.
  It primarily affects women in their early 50s and has a 10-year survival rate of 50% to 60%.

- *Invasive lobular carcinoma* tends to be multicentric, and bilateral in 30% of women. It accounts for 5% to 10% of all breast cancers. It primarily affects women in their 50s and has a 10-year survival rate of 50% to 60%.

- *Tubular carcinoma* is uncommon, occurring in only 2% of all women with breast cancer. It is a well-differentiated adenocarcinoma that occurs primarily in women over age 55. Microcalcifications are often present.

- *Medullary carcinoma* accounts for 5% to 7% of all breast cancers. It primarily affects women under age 55, and lymph node involvement is present in 40% of patients at diagnosis. It tends to be well circumscribed and bilateral, with a rapid growth rate.

- *Mucinous (colloid) carcinomas* are uncommon, representing only 3% of all breast cancers. They primarily affect women 60 to 70 years of age. The tumor tends to be bulky and slow growing.

- Other malignant tumors of the breast include sarcomas, invasive cribriform, papillary carcinoma, Paget's disease, and inflammatory breast cancer.

Patterns of Metastasis

Breast cancer metastasizes primarily to the bone, lungs, nodes, liver, and brain. Women with estrogen receptor–negative disease typically experience recurrence in visceral organs, whereas women with estrogen receptor–positive disease more often have recurrence in skin and bone.

Clinical Manifestations

- Boundaries of the mass are not distinct, lacking mobility due to tumor infiltration of adjacent tissues.
- Pain is not common in early disease.
- Pink or bloody, spontaneous, unilateral discharge may occur from the nipple.
- Tumor fixation or infiltration causes nipple elevation or retraction.
- Skin dimpling or retraction may occur due to invasion of suspensory ligaments and fixation to the chest wall.
- Heat and erythema may signify inflammatory breast cancer.
- Skin edema (peau d'orange) may be caused by tumor invasion and obstruction of dermal lymphatics.
- Ulceration of the skin with secondary infection
- Isolated skin nodules signify tumor invasion of blood vessels and lymphatics.
- Ulceration or scaly skin at the nipple may indicate Paget's disease.
- Early symptoms of liver involvement include loss of appetite and abnormal liver function tests, and indicate metastasis.
- Pulmonary involvement (metastases) may be manifested as nonproductive cough or shortness of breath. Pleural effusions may progress slowly over time.
- Metastasis to the brain or meningeal carcinomatosis may present as seizures or cranial nerve palsies.

Assessment

Diagnostic Procedures

Screening mammograms are used for routine observation of breast tissue. The goal is to detect malignancy before it becomes clinically apparent. Screening mammograms are recommended as a baseline at age 35, every 1 to 2 years for women aged 40 to 49, and yearly for women aged 50 and older.

A *diagnostic mammogram* is done when a patient reports symptoms, when clinical findings are suspicious, or when a screening mammogram reveals an abnormality. Information learned on diagnostic mammography may prevent the need for open biopsy.

A *sonogram* or *ultrasound* determines whether a lesion is solid or cystic. They are not as sensitive as a mammogram, but because they pose no danger to the developing fetus, they may be used in pregnant women.

Magnetic resonance imaging (MRI) may detect lesions early because it can determine smaller lesions and finer detail. It helps to distinguish benign from malignant lesions, avoiding benign biopsy.

Positron emission tomography (PET) employs metabolic activity to image the breast tissue. It may be able to differentiate between benign and malignant disease.

Fine-needle aspiration is used when an abnormality is known to be solid or to determine whether a lump is cystic. Surgical biopsy may still be necessary if the lesion is clinically suspicious.

Stereotactic needle-guided biopsy is most often used to target and identify nonpalpable lesions detected on mammography. It permits diagnosis of benign disease without the trauma or scarring related to open biopsy.

Wire localization biopsy is used to assist in the location of nonpalpable lesions for excisional biopsy.

Open biopsy is used to remove a lump or identified area along with a small amount of surrounding normal tissue.

Classification and Staging

Once a diagnosis of breast cancer is made, a complete evaluation of the disease is initiated to establish the stage of disease and the approach to treatment. Breast cancer is staged clinically based on the primary tumor characteristics, physical examination of axillary nodes, and presence of distant metastases.

- Stage I is tumor 0 to 2 cm in size; negative lymph nodes and no evidence of metastasis.
- Stage II represents a small tumor with positive lymph nodes or a larger tumor with negative nodes.
- Stage III is more advanced locoregional disease with no distant metastasis.
- Stage IV involves the presence of distant metastasis.

Treatment

Primary Breast Cancer
Surgery

- Lobular carcinoma tends to be bilateral and multicentric. If not treated, there is a 50% chance of invasive breast cancer developing in either breast.
  - Management includes observation with annual mammography and frequent physical examination, ipsilateral mastectomy with contralateral biopsy, or bilateral mastectomy with immediate or delayed reconstruction.
- Intraductal carcinoma rarely carries a risk of axillary node involvement.
  - Management includes total mastectomy with low axillary dissection, wide excision followed by radiation, or wide excision alone with tumor-free margins.
- Most women with stage I and stage II breast cancer with positive or negative nodes are treated by breast conservation procedures, in-

PART VI

cluding lumpectomy, partial mastectomy, segmental resection, or quadrantectomy and breast radiation.

- Invasive breast cancer requires level I and II axillary node dissection for staging purposes; sentinel node biopsy may be adequate to determine the need for adjuvant chemotherapy without axillary node dissection.

- Women who require chemotherapy because of the characteristics of their tumor in the absence of palpable axillary nodes may not require an axillary node dissection, because information gained would not add to the decision-making process.

- Modified radical mastectomy involves removal of all breast tissue and nipple–areola complex and level I and II axillary node dissection, and is indicated in the following circumstances:

  - Women with larger, multicentric tumors where adequate resection would not be possible with a lumpectomy alone

  - Women who prefer not to undergo radiation therapy, which would be mandatory with lumpectomy

  - Definitive treatment if disease should recur following conservative surgery and radiation therapy

Chemotherapy

Adjuvant chemotherapy is indicated for early stage I and II breast cancer as well as for larger, more poorly differentiated breast cancers. Adjuvant chemotherapy is indicated because

- metastatic disease occurs in 30% to 50% of women with node-negative breast cancer and

- the rate of disease recurrence in node-negative disease can be reduced 20% to 50% by adjuvant therapy.

Potential drug combinations

- Methotrexate, followed in 1 hour by 5-fluoro-uracil (M-F); leucovorin calcium (L) is given beginning 24 hours after administration of methotrexate.

  - The regimen is given on days 1 and 8, every 28 days for 6 cycles. There is minimal myelo-suppression, gonadal dysfunction, and hair loss.

- Cyclophosphamide, methotrexate, and 5-fluorouracil (CMF)

  - Methotrexate and 5-fluorouracil are given on days 1 and 8; cyclophosphamide is given orally for 14 days; CMF combination is administered every 28 days for 6 cycles.

  - Myelosuppression, hair loss, and gonadal dysfunction are more pronounced with this regimen.

- Doxorubicin and cyclophosphamide (AC), given in standard doses every 3 weeks for 4 cycles.

  - This is a treatment option for women with high-risk, node-negative disease or with node-positive disease.

  - The taxanes (docetaxel and paclitaxel) are often given in combination with AC for women with more advanced disease.

  - Herceptin may also be given in the above combination in women who are positive for the *HER-2* gene.

- Treatment with tamoxifen is based on patient age (over 50) and estrogen receptor status. It may be given alone or in combination with chemotherapy.

- Goserelin acetate (luteinizing hormone–releasing hormone antagonist), with or without tamoxifen and chemotherapy, may be used to treat premenopausal women with estrogen receptor–positive, node-positive disease.

PART VI

Radiation

If radiation is indicated, it generally begins 3 to 4 weeks after chemotherapy is complete. Skin changes and arm swelling may occur. If chemotherapy is given along with radiation, chemotherapy should be held until the skin heals.

Breast Reconstruction

Breast reconstruction is often undertaken at the time of mastectomy or shortly after chemotherapy is complete. The ideal candidate is the woman with early-stage disease, no nodal involvement, and low risk factors for recurrence. Women who are pregnant or breastfeeding, or who have tissue abnormalities, infection, lupus, scleroderma, or uncontrolled diabetes, are not candidates. Those with radiation damage, vascularization problems, or who have inadequate tissue available are not eligible.

- Silicone implants
  - Silicone implants are used when there is adequate skin for coverage after mastectomy.
  - The ideal candidate is small-breasted and has a minimum of ptosis on the contralateral breast.
  - An incision is made in the previous scar and a pocket is made beneath the chest wall muscles, where the silicone implant is placed.
  - Complications include contracture, infection, hematoma, and flap necrosis.
- Saline tissue expanders
  - Saline tissue expanders are used when there is inadequate supply of skin after mastectomy or when the breast is large and/or ptotic.
  - An expander is placed behind the muscles of the chest wall using the lines of the mastectomy incision.
  - The filling port is injected with saline over 6 to 8 weeks until the device is overinflated by

50%; it is left overinflated for several months to allow for stretching and more natural contour.

- The expander is removed after several months and replaced with a permanent prosthesis.

- Latissimus dorsi flap
  - This flap is used when adequate skin is not available at the mastectomy site and/or if additional tissue is needed to fill the supraclavicular hollow and create an anterior axillary fold after mastectomy.

- Transverse rectus abdominis muscle flap, or "tummy tuck"
  - Involves an incision over the lower abdomen; abdominal muscle and fat are tunneled under abdominal skin to the mastectomy site. Complications include hernia at the donor site and flap necrosis. Obese patients, patients with circulatory problems, smokers, and patients over 65 are not candidates.

- Nipple areolar construction
  - Accomplished by using tissue from the opposite breast or from like tissue on the inner thigh or postauricular area. Tattooing may be necessary to darken the skin.

Breast Cancer in Men

Breast cancer in men is similar to the same disease in women in terms of epidemiology, natural history, treatment options, and response to treatment.

- It occurs most commonly in men aged 50 to 70 years, and most are estrogen receptor–positive.

- It typically presents as infiltrating ductal carcinoma, fixed to the underlying fascia and skin; nipple retraction and bloody discharge may be present.

- Because it is usually first diagnosed at an advanced stage, prognosis is generally poor.

PART VI

- Treatment is usually by modified radical mastectomy.
- Hormonal manipulation is indicated, using tamoxifen, Arimidex, or Zoladex, unless the disease is life-threatening or aggressive, indicating the use of chemotherapy.

Metastatic Breast Cancer

Metastatic breast cancer is present at clinical diagnosis in approximately 10% of women. Thirty percent to 40% of women treated and presumed to be cured actually have metastatic disease, which recurs usually within 2 years of diagnosis despite systemic therapy. Median survival for patients with stage IV disease is 2 to 3 years.

Management of metastatic breast cancer involves judicious use of both local and systemic measures to palliate symptoms and improve the patient's quality of life. The initial therapy is generally the one that is least toxic with the highest response rate.

Chemotherapy

- Candidates include women whose disease is hormone receptor–negative, who are refractory to hormone therapy, or who have aggressive disease in the liver or pulmonary system.
- Most chemotherapy regimens include some combination of methotrexate, 5-fluorouracil, cyclophosphamide, doxorubicin, paclitaxel, docetaxel, vinorelbine, doxorubicon HCL, or epirubicin. If the patient is *HER-2* positive, Herceptin as a single agent would be indicated as a first-line agent because it has minimal toxicity.

Endocrine Therapy

- Hormone manipulation is the main treatment for women with metastatic breast cancer that is estrogen receptor–positive.
- Steroid hormones promote tumor growth in hormonally dependent breast cancer; therefore,

surgical removal of the hormone source or medical manipulation of hormone balance results in significant tumor regression, but not cure.

- Antiestrogen therapy
  - Tamoxifen is the most widely used antiestrogen. If the woman has been on tamoxifen and experienced recurrence, the tamoxifen would be stopped and another form of hormone manipulation would be given.
  - Side effects of tamoxifen are minimal, including hot flashes, mild nausea, fluid retention and ankle swelling, vaginal cornification, and postmenopausal bleeding.
  - Other antiestrogens include toremifene and raloxifene, with similar efficacy to that of tamoxifen.
- Aromatase inhibitors
  - Aromatase inhibitors (e.g., anastrozole, letrozole, or exemestane) are shown to be therapeutic in metastatic breast cancer.
- Progestin therapy
  - Megestrol acetate is a progesterone agent that is tolerated as well as tamoxifen and has comparable efficacy.
- Oophorectomy
  - Oophorectomy is generally reserved for women with recurrent or metastatic disease, if disease is not life-threatening at the time of recurrence. Zoladex injections may be used instead of an oophorectomy, because they essentially create a medical oophorectomy. The effect of zoladex is not as immediate as that of oophorectomy.
  - Surgical oophorectomy, tamoxifen, or ovarian radiation are equally effective in removing endogenous estrogen sources in premenopausal women and in some perimenopausal women.

PART VI

Supportive Care

Bone Metastasis

- Bone pain may occur before skeletal changes are seen on radiography; a bone scan is a sensitive method to detect metastatic disease.
- CA 15-3, a human breast tumor–associated antigen, is a sensitive marker in breast cancer metastases and may be used as a screening test for bone metastases.
- Metastasis to bone marrow is indicated by anemia, thrombocytopenia, leukocytosis, and immature forms of nucleated red blood cells; serum alkaline phosphatase and serum calcium levels may be increased.
- Patients who have back pain should undergo a thorough neurological examination and radiographic evaluation of the spine; MRI may determine whether spinal cord compression is present or imminent.
- Radiation to symptomatic areas often results in effective pain relief and bone recalcification.
- Surgery may stabilize bone by internal fixation or replacement to avoid impending fracture.
- Bisphosphonates (etidronate, clodronate, pamidronate) are used to inhibit bone demineralization and to reduce incidence of bone pain, hypercalcemia, and even metastatic disease progression in bone; treatment is usually monthly.

Spinal Cord Compression

- This condition constitutes an emergency because of the potential for paraplegia; pain is usually present for several weeks before other neurological symptoms develop.
- It may be secondary to epidural tumor or altered bone alignment because of pathological fracture.
- Imminent compression should be suspected in those with known bone disease; progressive back pain is associated with weakness, pares-

thesias, bowel or bladder dysfunction, or gait disturbances.

- MRI should be done as soon as the diagnosis is suspected to determine the exact level of compression and to identify other occult extradural lesions.
- Optimal results and return to ambulation can be accomplished by combined therapy with radiotherapy and corticosteroids.
- When spinal cord compression develops and diagnosis of epidural metastasis is in doubt, or if the patient's neurological state worsens as radiotherapy progresses, decompression laminectomy may be performed.

Brain Metastasis and Leptomeningeal Carcinomatosis

- Brain metastasis occurs in approximately 30% of women with breast cancer and generally presents as headache, motor weakness, seizures, and mental and visual changes.
- Symptoms of brain metastasis can be managed by gamma knife, total-brain irradiation, and corticosteroids.
- The most common signs of leptomeningeal carcinomatosis are headache, cranial nerve dysfunction, and changes in mental status.
- Treatment is with total-brain irradiation, followed by intraventricular–intrathecal chemotherapy, usually through an Ommaya reservoir.

Chronic Lymphedema

- Occurs most commonly in women who have undergone axillary dissection followed by radiation therapy
- Most often caused by infection and tumor recurrence or tumor enlargement in axilla
- Management techniques: elevation of the arm, elastic stockinette wraps, therapeutic massage, weight loss, and weight control.

Chapter 38

Central Nervous System Cancers

<u>BRAIN TUMORS</u>

Incidence

Cancer of the central nervous system (CNS) includes primary and metastatic tumors of the brain and spinal cord. CNS tumors are associated with a significant degree of morbidity and mortality. Primary CNS cancers represent approximately 2% of cancers. Malignant CNS tumors are responsible for 2.5% of cancer-related deaths.

The peak incidence of brain tumors occurs in the first, fifth, sixth, and seventh decades. An increasing incidence of primary brain tumors has been noted in the elderly. In children, brain cancer is the second most common cancer diagnosed.

Etiology

Genetic Disorders
- Neurofibromatosis type 1 is an autosomal dominant disorder associated with optic nerve gliomas, astrocytomas, ependymomas, and meningiomas.
- Li-Fraumeni syndrome and Turcot syndrome are both autosomal dominant disorders associated with an increased incidence of gliomas, medulloblastomas, and pituitary adenomas.
- Recent advances in molecular biology have identified both the expression of activated oncogenes and the inactivation of tumor-suppressor genes in a variety of brain tumors. Epidermal growth factor receptor has been found to be amplified in glioblastoma patients.

Chemical and Environmental Factors

- Workers exposed to chemicals in pesticides, herbicides, and fertilizers have had a higher than expected incidence of gliomas.
- Synthetic rubber, petrochemicals, industrial chemicals, and nuclear energy have been associated with gliomas.

Viral Factors

- Patients with AIDS and primary CNS lymphomas (PCNSLs) have a higher rate of infection with the Epstein-Barr virus.
- Individuals with human immunodeficiency virus (HIV) have an increased risk for developing PCNSL.

Radiation

- Radiation to the head has been linked to subsequent brain tumors and has been noted to be a factor in the higher than usual incidence of brain tumors in children treated for acute lymphoblastic leukemia and tinea capitis.

Electromagnetic Fields

- Epidemiological studies have suggested a possible association between exposure to electromagnetic fields and increased incidence of cancers, specifically gliomas.

Pathophysiology

Types of CNS Tumors

Gliomas

- *Astrocytomas* occur most often in the fifth and sixth decades of life and account for 60% of all primary brain tumors. They generally arise in the cerebral hemispheres and range from well differentiated to highly malignant.
- *Oligodendrogliomas* account for 5% of primary brain tumors and are usually located in the frontal lobe. They tend to be slow growing and commonly present as a seizure disorder.

- *Glioblastomas* are high-grade astrocytomas with a necrotic component. They generally arise in the cerebral hemispheres during the fifth and sixth decades of life.

Primary Central Nervous System Lymphomas

- PCNSLs are increasing, with the highest incidence occurring in patients with AIDS, in which PCNSL develops in up to 6% of cases.
- PCNSLs commonly involve the frontal lobes and disseminate within the CNS and eyes.
- They generally present with lethargy, confusion, apathy, headache, nausea, vomiting, hemiparesis, visual disturbances, and seizures.

Metastatic Brain Tumors

- Twenty percent to 40% of patients with systemic cancer develop brain metastases, and this number is increasing as patients live longer.
- Brain metastases occur at three sites: the brain parenchyma, the skull and dura, and the leptomeninges.
- Symptoms include headache, nausea, vomiting, change in level of consciousness, diminished cognitive function, personality changes, hemiparesis, language problems, and seizures.
- Meningeal carcinomatosis from an adenocarcinoma of breast, lung, gastrointestinal tract, melanoma, and childhood leukemia occurs in approximately 4% of cases.

Clinical Manifestations

Increased Intracranial Pressure

Clinical manifestations of brain tumors occur because they create a mass effect and increase intracranial pressure (ICP). Clinical manifestations produced by the effects of increasing pressure on nerve cells, blood vessels, and dura include

- mental changes,
- papilledema,

- headache,
- vomiting,
- changes in vital signs, and
- hemiparesis or hemiplegia.

Focal Effects
Focal effects are caused by direct compression of nerve tissue or destruction and invasion of brain tissues; deficits are directly related to the affected area of the brain. Focal or generalized seizures are major symptoms of brain tumors and are the first clinical manifestation of a brain tumor in many adults.

Patients with metastatic brain tumors commonly have headache first, followed by focal weakness, mental disturbances, and seizures; aphasia and visual abnormalities also may occur.

Displacement of Brain Structure
As brain structures become displaced by shifting brain tissues, compression damage, cerebral edema, and ischemia cause effects that may be irreversible. Herniation of brain tissue can occur.

- Supratentorial herniations cause changes in level of consciousness and inocular, motor, and respiratory signs.
- Infratentorial herniations cause loss of consciousness and changes in cardiac and respiratory signs.

Assessment
A complete neurological assessment involves evaluation of both focal and generalized symptoms. Each symptom is evaluated with regard to location, onset, and duration of the symptom. Baseline measures of neurological function are noted.

Diagnostic Measures
Computerized tomography (CT) views one plane of the cranium over a few seconds. Photographs

PART VI

give the exact location and size of nodules as well as surrounding edema. CT is less costly, compared with MRI.

Magnetic resonance imaging (MRI) allows multiplane imaging and provides information regarding histology and pathology of lesions and extent of tissue invasion, depth of lesions, the presence of cysts, the amount of edema surrounding a tumor, and the presence of calcium aggregates.

Positron emission tomography (PET) combines properties of conventional nuclear scanning with physical characteristics of positron-emitting radionuclides. It provides information about tumor metabolism, blood flow, and oxygen and glucose use.

Classification and Staging

Clinical staging is based on neurological signs and symptoms and on results of diagnostic tests. The most important feature in the classification of CNS tumors is histopathology. Pathological staging is based on results of histopathological studies, tumor grade, and microscopic evidence of completeness of tumor resection.

Treatment

Surgery

Surgery is the primary treatment for resectable primary brain tumors and some isolated metastatic lesions. Surgery is a treatment option based on tumor location, tumor size, method of tumor spread, and the patient's neurological status and general health.

Goals of surgery

- Establish a diagnosis by providing tissue for histological examination.
- Provide relief of symptoms by quickly reducing the tumor bulk.
- Alleviate ICP and the mass effect caused by compression or infiltration of brain tissue.
- Decreasing the tumor burden may increase the

effectiveness of adjuvant therapy as well as provide room for edema that may develop with radiation therapy.

Complications of surgery include intracranial bleeding, cerebral edema, water intoxication, decreased level of consciousness, increased ICP, progressive hemiparesis, signs of herniation, and seizures.

Radiosurgery
- Stereotactic radiosurgery is a noninvasive technique that delivers a single large fraction of ionizing radiation to a small, well-defined intracranial target. This technique is performed using a modified linear accelerator (gamma knife).
- A laser is used to vaporize the tumor. This procedure is especially effective in the treatment of tumors in or near sensitive target structures.

Radiotherapy
- Radiotherapy is used for both primary and metastatic disease; response is based on cell type and tissue of origin.
- Corticosteroid therapy may be needed to relieve cerebral swelling and promote improvement of symptoms.
- The presence of hypoxic malignant cells limits the effectiveness of radiation therapy.
- Administration of intraoperative radiation may help to shield normal tissue from radiation effects while exposing the tumor to maximum radiation effects.
- Three-dimensional conformal radiation therapy is a method of high-precision radiation therapy using CT information. The radiation dose is delivered to conform to the anatomical boundaries of the tumor.

Chemotherapy and Biotherapy
- Most chemotherapeutic agents do not cross the blood–brain barrier. Nitrosoureas are drugs that

are lipid soluble and can penetrate the blood–brain barrier. Intraarterial, intrathecal, and intratumoral drug delivery may circumvent the blood–brain barrier.

- Certain chemotherapeutic agents are used to enhance the effect of radiation (e.g., 5-fluoro-uracil, BCNU).

- Chemotherapy is indicated for histologic grade III or grade IV tumors.

Supportive Care

General supportive care to prepare the family and the home environment for the patient who is suffering from any degree of physical or mental impairment requires intensive planning and consultation between home care agencies and the health care team. Often patients will need to be stabilized in the hospital and transferred to the home or a care facility where the physical as well as emotional needs may be addressed.

- Cerebral edema is generally managed with corticosteroids to reduce the edema over a period of hours or days.

- Osmotherapy is used to reduce the amount of fluid in brain tissue. Hyperosmolor agents such as mannitol are administered intravenously, and fluid intake is restricted.

- Increased ICP is managed by elevating the head of the bed, avoiding head rotation, neck flexion, and extension. Efforts are made to avoid the Valsalva maneuver, isometric muscle contractions, and emotional arousal. Sneezing, coughing, and straining, as well as lying in the prone position, may aggravate any ICP.

- Seizures may occur as a result of compression by the tumor, and the patient's safety is at risk. Prophylactic anticonvulsant medication is appropriate. Providing a safe environment and providing for skin and oral hygiene after a seizure are important nursing measures.

SPINAL CORD TUMORS

Incidence
Primary spinal cord tumors account for only 15% of all primary CNS tumors. They occur most often in persons age 20 to 60. Metastatic tumors are much more common than primary spinal cord tumors.

Etiology
The etiology of primary spinal cord tumors is unknown. Individuals with NF-1 may develop neurofibromas of the spinal cord, spinal nerve root tumors may be present in those with NF-2, and individuals with von Hippel-Lindau disease are at risk for developing spinal hemangioblastomas.

Pathophysiology

Extradural Tumors
Extradural tumors lie outside the dura. Most are metastatic cancers to the vertebral column, originating from the breast, lung, prostate, kidney, and multiple myeloma.

- Most tumors to the spinal cord compress the cord anteriorly, leading to edema and ischemia of the spinal cord, and mechanically distort and damage the nerve tissue.
- The thoracic spine is the most frequent location of epidural spinal cord compression, followed by the lumbosacral and cervical spine.

Intradural Tumors
Intradural tumors arise from the nerve roots or coverings of the spinal cord or develop in the spinal cord itself. Schwannomas are the most common extramedullary tumor, followed by meningiomas. Approximately 50% of spinal cord tumors are located in the thoracic spine, 30% are located in the lumbosacral region, and 20% involve the cervical spine.

PART VI

Clinical Manifestations

Extramedullary tumors affect the cord by compression of the spinal nerve root, displacement of the spinal cord itself, interference with the spinal blood supply, or obstruction of cerebrospinal fluid (CSF) circulation. The signs and symptoms of spinal cord tumors are pain, motor weakness, sensory impairment, and autonomic dysfunction involving the bowel and bladder.

Assessment

Diagnostic Studies

MRI is the diagnostic procedure of choice for the evaluation of both intramedullary and extramedullary spinal cord tumors.

Treatment

Surgery is the initial treatment for intramedullary tumors and some extradural tumors. A laminectomy decompresses the spinal cord, and the spinal column is stabilized anteriorly, often with Steinmann pins or plates. Patients with spinal instability due to tumor invasion must undergo a stabilization procedure or be fitted for a brace.

Complications related to the surgical intervention include standard surgical risks as well as the development of neurological deficits. A CSF leak may develop because the dura is not completely sealed or a tear was not allowed to heal.

Radiation involves delivery of doses of 45 to 50 Gy in 180-cGy fractions. Steroids are also given, especially if there is neurological dysfunction. Radiation myelopathy results from demyelination of the spinal cord over time. Paresthesias or numbness occurs over a 3- to 4-month period following treatment and generally resolves within 3 to 6 months.

Chapter 39

Cervical Cancer

Incidence

Cervical cancer is a significant cause of morbidity and mortality worldwide. Annually, approximately 12,800 new cases and 4800 deaths from cervical cancer occur in the United States. Mortality has decreased in women over age 45 but has increased in women under age 35.

Overall incidence of invasive cancer has decreased as a result of the Pap smear, yet incidence of carcinoma in situ (CIS) has increased. Women in their 20s are most often diagnosed with cervical dysplasia, women aged 30 to 39 are most often diagnosed with CIS, and women over age 40 are most often diagnosed with invasive cancer.

Etiology

Many personal risk factors have been associated with precancerous lesions of the cervix.

- Low socioeconomic group
- Smoking
- Early sexual activity (before age 17)
- Multiple sexual partners
- Multiparous
- Work in manufacturing, personal services, farm work, or as a nurse's aide
- Sexually transmitted infections
- Human immunodeficiency virus (HIV)
- Herpes simplex virus type 2
- Human papillomavirus
- In utero exposure to diethylstilbestrol
- Spouse whose previous wife had cervical cancer

PART VI

- Spouse with early sexual activity, multiple partners
- Spouse with cancer of penis
- African American or Hispanic origin

Certain behaviors may actually lower the risk of cervical cancer.

- Barrier-type contraception
- Vasectomy
- Recommended daily allowances of vitamins A and C and beta carotene
- Limited number of sexual partners
- Sexual activity initiated at later age

Pathophysiology

Cellular Characteristics
Histologically, 80% to 90% of cervical tumors are squamous cell tumors. The remainder are mostly adenocarcinoma.

Progression of Disease
Cervical cancer is a progressive disease that begins with neoplastic alteration of cells at the squamocolumnar junction (premalignant disease) and gradually progresses to involve the epithelium and invade the stroma (invasive disease).

Patterns of Spread
Once invasive, cervical cancer spreads by four routes:

1. *Direct extension* throughout the entire cervix, into the parametrium, uterus, bladder, and rectum
2. *Lymphatic,* which includes the obturator, hypogastric, external iliac, and then the parametrial, presacral, and inferior gluteal nodes
3. *Hematogenous* through the venous plexus and paracervical veins
4. *Intraperitoneal implantation*

The most common sites for metastases are lung, liver, bone, and mediastinal and supraclavicular nodes.

Classification and Staging

The Bethesda System is typically used to report cervical cytological diagnosis from Pap smears and includes the following descriptors:

- Adequacy of cytologic specimen
- General categorization of diagnosis (normal, abnormal)
- Descriptive diagnosis (atypical cells, low grade, high grade, etc.)

Cervical Intraepithelial Neoplasia or Squamous Intraepithelial Lesions

Cervical intraepithelial neoplasia (CIN) and *squamous intraepithelial lesion (SIL)* are two terms used in the classification of progression of the disease process. CIN is divided into three categories—CIN I, CIN II, and CIN III—which describe progression of disease and whether disease is considered invasive or malignant. Low-grade or high-grade SIL describes cellular changes.

- CIN I or low-grade SIL indicates dysplasia or atypical changes involving less than one-third thickness of the epithelium.
- CIN II or high-grade SIL indicates dysplasia involving two-thirds thickness of the epithelium.
- CIN III or high-grade SIL indicates severe dysplasia or CIS and involves up to full thickness of the epithelium.
- CIN III is more likely to progress than is CIN I or II; there is no way to predict which will progress.
- Invasive disease is malignant disease that extends beyond the basement membrane.

PART VI

Staging

Staging is based on clinical findings, with confirmation from examination completed under anesthesia. Initial staging is one of the best prognostic indicators.

Approximate 5-year survival rates

- Stage I: 85%
- Stage II: 60%
- Stage III: 25% to 50%
- Stage IV: < 10%

Clinical Manifestations

In preinvasive and early stages, cervical cancer is asymptomatic except for watery vaginal discharge.

Late disease symptoms

- Postcoital bleeding
- Intermenstrual bleeding
- Heavy menstrual flow
- Symptoms related to anemia
- Foul-smelling, serous vaginal discharge
- Pain in pelvis, hypogastrium, flank, leg
- Urinary or rectal symptoms

End-stage disease may be characterized by

- edema of the lower extremities,
- massive vaginal hemorrhage, and
- renal failure.

Diagnostic Measures

For SILs, the typical diagnostic measure is the Pap smear. The Pap smear is the most effective tool for assessing and diagnosing preinvasive disease and cervical cancer.

- A Pap smear is recommended annually for all sexually active women or for those over 18 years of age; a pelvic examination also should be done.

- Frequency of examinations may be altered by the individual's physician.

If the Pap smear shows CIN or SIL, the next steps in diagnosis are

- clinical examination under anesthesia,
- cervical biopsy,
- endocervical curettage,
- cystoscopy,
- proctosigmoidoscopy, and
- metastatic work-up (chest x-ray, intravenous pyelogram, barium enema, hematological profile, liver scan, CT or MRI, node biopsies, and DNA subtyping).

Treatment

Accurate evaluation of extent of disease before treatment is critical. Treatment for CIN or SIL varies greatly from that for invasive disease.

CIN or SIL

Treatment is based on the extent of disease and on the woman's desire to preserve reproductive function.

Treatment options

- Cervical biopsy
- Electrocautery
- Cryosurgery
  - Most commonly used method
  - Painless
  - Low morbidity
  - Outpatient procedure
  - Patients experience watery discharge for 2 to 4 weeks.
- Laser surgery
  - 80% to 90% of CIN or SIL can be eradicated.
  - Less disease-free tissue removed
  - Slight discomfort

- Little vaginal discharge
- Heals in 2 to 3 weeks
- Electrosurgery: loop diathermy excision (LEEP)
  - Outpatient surgery, general anesthesia
  - Minimal tissue ablation
  - Slight discharge
- Cone biopsy
  - Removes cone-shaped piece of tissue from endocervix and exocervix
  - Diagnostic or therapeutic
  - Potential hemorrhage or perforation
  - Delayed complications include bleeding, cervical stenosis, and infertility.
- Hysterectomy for high-grade SIL (CIN III)
  - May be used for treatment of women who have completed childbearing

Invasive Disease

Treatment is based on a woman's age, medical condition, and extent of disease. Either surgery or radiation can be used equally effectively for patients with early-stage disease. In general, stages IIb to IV are initially treated with radiotherapy. Treatment selection is related to stage of disease.

Stage IA (Microinvasive)

- Hysterectomy: abdominal or vaginal, for women who do not desire childbearing
- Conization for patients who are poor surgical risks or prefer to preserve fertility

Stages IB and IIA

Treatment selection is controversial; choice is often based on the oncologist's experiences.

- Radical abdominal hysterectomy and pelvic lymphadenectomy: ovarian function preserved; vagina more pliable than with radiation; shorter treatment time
- Definitive radiation with external beam radiotherapy and/or intracavitary insertion

Stages IIB, III, and IVA

High-dose external beam radiation followed by brachytherapy

- Outpatient therapy
- Eliminates need for surgery
- Suitable for poor surgical candidates

Pretreatment staging laparotomy

- Can identify candidates for specific therapies but is plagued by complications and minimal improvement in survival
- Alternative: extraperitoneal exploration for staging

Pelvic exenteration

- Used only in selected patients previously treated with radiation, who have recurrent centralized disease not adherent to pelvic side walls or involving lymph nodes
- Inoperable disease found in about 60% of cases

Recurrent or Persistent Disease

About 35% of women have recurrent or persistent disease. Follow-up is critical, though recurrence is difficult to detect. Survival averages 6 to 10 months. Most recurrences (80%) occur within 2 years of therapy.

Signs of recurrence

- Unexplained weight loss
- Leg edema
- Pain in pelvis or thigh
- Serosanguineous vaginal discharge
- Cough, hemoptysis, chest pain
- The triad of weight loss, leg edema, and pelvic pain has a grim outlook.

Most treatment is palliative, and control is rare. Treatments include surgery, radiation therapy, and chemotherapy.

Surgery

Pelvic exenteration may be considered for central recurrence. Only a small number of women with recurrence are candidates for this procedure.

Radiotherapy

May be used to treat metastatic disease outside initial radiation field; selectively used within previously irradiated fields.

Chemotherapy

This treatment modality is complicated by decreased pelvic vascular perfusion, limited bone marrow reserve, and poor renal function. Response rates range from 0% to 48%, with no long-term benefit. Response rates are higher in patients with no prior chemotherapy or radiation.

Chemotherapeutic agents

- Cisplatin has the greatest single-agent activity.
- Carboplatin may be used as first-line therapy.
- Other agents include doxorubicin, dibromodulcitol, ifosfamide, gemcitabine, and topotecan.
- Combination agents are not more effective than single agents.
- Chemotherapy can be used as radiosensitizer, particularly hydroxyurea or cisplatin.

Supportive Care

Major nursing management issues

- Education of the patient
- Management of treatment-induced complications and side effects
- Counseling on sexuality issues and concerns
- Assessment of response and anticipation of recurrence

Chapter 40

Colorectal Cancer

Incidence
Colorectal cancer is the third most commonly occurring cancer and the third leading cause of
death from cancer for both men and women.
There are an estimated 131,000 new cases each
year and 55,000 deaths each year resulting from
colorectal cancer. Incidence is higher in industrialized regions where diets are high in fats and
proteins and low in vegetable and fruit content.
Peak incidence is in the sixth and seventh
decades. Overall 5-year survival rate is 90% for
disease diagnosed in the early stage and 60% for
advanced stages.

Etiology
There are many risk factors associated with colorectal cancer:

- Age (people 50 years or older)
- Dietary factors appear to have dominant role.
  - Fat increases the risk of colon cancer
  - High-fiber diets may decrease the effects of
    fatty acids, increase fecal bulk and stool tran-
    sit time, and hence reduce potential carcino-
    genic action.
- Alcohol consumption, particularly beer and
  whiskey
- Genetics: a family history of
  - familial adenomatous polyposis,
  - hereditary nonpolyposis colon cancer,
  - Gardner's, Turcot, and Peutz-Jeghers syn-
    dromes, and
  - colorectal cancer.
- Inflammatory bowel conditions

PART VI

- Ulcerative colitis
- Crohn's disease
- Radiation therapy to pelvis
- Ureterosigmoidostomy leads to increased risk 15 years after surgery.

Prevention
Preventive measures
- Decreased fat intake
- Increased intake of fruits and vegetables
- Total daily fiber intake of 20 to 30 grams
- Use of antioxidants (beta carotene, vitamin C, vitamin E, calcium)
- Use of nonsteroidal antiinflammatory drugs

Screening techniques
- Fecal occult blood test
- At age 40, digital rectal examination
- After age 50, annual examination, fecal occult blood, and flexible sigmoidoscopy every 3 to 5 years
- If at high risk, colonoscopy is recommended, and screening should occur every year.

Pathophysiology
Adenocarcinoma is the most common histological type. The most common anatomic sites affected are the descending and sigmoid colon. Progression of disease does not relate to symptoms. Colon cancer develops first in the mucosa and will invade locally by direct extension. Submucosal involvement leads to lymph and vascular spread. Liver is the most common site of metastases, but it can also metastasize to bone, brain, kidneys, and adrenals.

Clinical Manifestations
Manifestations of colorectal cancer correlate to the location of the tumor.

Signs and symptoms
- Early stage: asymptomatic, abdominal pain, and flatulence
- Late stage: severe pain, anorexia, weight loss, jaundice, ascites, and hepatomegaly
- Tumors of descending/sigmoid colon
  - Constipation alternating with diarrhea
  - Obstruction (nausea/vomiting)
  - Abdominal pain
  - Melena
  - Perforation
- Tumors in ascending colon
  - Vague abdominal aching
  - Weakness
  - Weight loss
  - Fatigue
  - Palpitations
  - Anemia
- Tumors of transverse colon
  - Constipation alternating with diarrhea
  - Melena
  - Bowel obstruction and pain
- Tumors of rectum
  - Bleeding with bright red blood
  - Sense of incomplete evacuation
  - Tenesmus, sense of fullness
  - Change in bowel movement
  - Pelvic pain
- Tumors of anus
  - Bleeding
  - Discharge
  - Rectal mass
  - Pain on defecation

Assessment
Physical examination is focused on specific gastrointestinal symptoms, prior medical and family

history, risk factors, digital examination of the rectal area, and vaginal examination for fistulas.

Diagnostic studies

- Carcinoembryonic antigen (CEA) and CA 19-9 levels
- Endoscopic examination; proctosigmoidoscopy
- Barium enema
- Fecal occult blood testing
- Hematological studies
- Chest x-ray
- CT scan
- DNA content analysis by flow cytometry
- Metastatic work-up: abdominal films and scans, liver function studies

Classification and Staging

Classification and staging is commonly done using a modified Dukes' and tumor-node-metastasis (TNM) system.

The prognosis with colorectal cancer is directly related to the stage at diagnosis.

- Prognosis for early stages I and II is favorable (90%).
- Prognosis for later stages (III and IV) is poor (60%).

Treatment

Surgery

Surgery is primary treatment for colorectal cancer. Adequate margins and complete excision provide the best outcomes.

Common surgical procedures

- Right hemicolectomy for tumors of the cecum, ascending colon, and hepatic flexure
- Transverse colectomy for tumors in the mid-transverse colon
- Left hemicolectomy for tumors of the left or descending colon

- Low anterior resection for tumors of the sigmoid colon and proximal rectum
- Subtotal colectomy for multiple synchronous tumors and distal transverse lesions
- Abdominal perineal resection for rectal tumors and more advanced disease

Complications of surgery, in addition to functional and anatomic alterations produced by surgery

- Anastomotic leak (pain, abscess, peritonitis)
- Intraabdominal abscess (fever, leukocytosis)
- Staphylococcal enteritis (diarrhea, sepsis)
- Obstruction (constipation, pain, nausea/vomiting)
- Genitourinary tract injury (leakage, oliguria, anuria)
- Sexual dysfunction (impotence)
- Ostomy complications (peristomal skin or stoma)

Radiation Therapy

Radiation therapy is used as adjuvant therapy to prevent local recurrence. Radiation can be used in preoperative, intraoperative, and postoperative treatment. The most common use of radiation is postoperatively.

Treatment considerations

- Preoperative radiation is given to decrease existing tumor burden and reduce the risk of local failure.
- Postoperative radiation is used for those at high risk of local recurrence.
- Both pre- and postoperative radiation (sandwich technique) can be used to decrease tumor dissemination.
- Palliative radiation controls advanced symptoms (pain, bleeding).
- Intraoperative radiation delivers a high dose directly to a localized area.

PART VI

Investigational radiation techniques used to enhance radiation effect

- Altered fractionation schemes
- Particle beam therapy
- Hyperthermia
- Brachytherapy
- Combinations of radiation and 5-FU

The most common side effects of radiation to the colorectal region are proctosigmoiditis, increased bowel motility, enteritis, fibrosis, stricture, and nausea and vomiting.

Chemotherapy

Chemotherapy targets the possible occult disease left after surgery and aims to reduce the risk of recurrence. Adjuvant therapy for stage I disease is not indicated, for stage II disease it is debatable, but for stage III and IV there are clear indications for chemotherapy.

Chemotherapeutic agents

- 5-Fluorouracil (5-FU), leukovorin, and levamisole is the most commonly used regimen.
- Irinotecan is being studied as second-line therapy for disease refractory to 5-FU.

Chemoradiation is the preferred treatment for anal cancers. 5-FU plus mitomycin and radiation is the standard approach.

Immunotherapy

Levamisole is an immunomodulator that enhances the effect of 5-FU as adjuvant therapy for stage III colon cancer. Interferon, interleukin-2, and bacillus Calmette-Guérin (BCG) are being studied extensively.

Supportive Care

There are several anticipated and unanticipated developments that can occur with colorectal cancer. The most common problems and approaches to care are discussed below.

Perineal Wound

Primary closure of the wound is the least complicated approach. Secondary closure prolongs the healing process and can take as along as 4 months. Packing and meticulous wound care are needed.

Bowel Obstruction

Although bowel obstruction may occur anytime, it is more common and develops more rapidly with advanced disease. Obstruction can occur from within the bowel lumen or from outside compression by invasive tumor growth. Signs and symptoms include nausea, unrelenting vomiting, abdominal pain, constipation, and absence of bowel sounds.

The usual treatment is nasogastric suction and intravenous fluids. A gastrostomy tube or PEG may be needed. Pharmacological management involves somatostatin, or ocreatide to minimize intestinal secretions.

Fistulas

Tumors may extend and create fistulous openings to the skin, vagina, and other organs. Treatments include stabilizing the fluid and electrolyte balance, preventing infection, and promoting spontaneous wound closure or using surgical resection or bypass of the fistulous tract.

Stoma and Colostomy Management

Care includes attention to stoma site selection, stoma management, and maintenance of gastrointestinal function. The stoma must be evaluated for viability, condition, size, shape, and whether sutures are holding the stoma onto the abdomen. Initially, there will be serosanguineous fluid draining from the stoma, which eventually evolves to normal stool secretions. Key principles in management are containment of the effluent and odor and protection of the peristomal skin.

PART VI

Sexual Dysfunction

The more extensive the surgery, the greater the potential for sexual dysfunction. Abdominoperineal resection has had the highest incidence of sexual problems: 65% of patients became sexually inactive, 50% were unable to ejaculate, and 45% reported erectile dysfunction. Removal of the rectum may interfere with the potential for orgasm.

Treatment approaches are specific to the underlying causes and may involve antidepressants, fatigue management, pain relief, odor control, and surgical measures to provide alternate sexual function.

Ureteral Obstruction

Obstruction occurs in 38% of patients and presents with oliguria and elevated serum creatinine level. Cystoscopy and retrograde pyelogram are used to diagnose obstruction. Urinary stents can be inserted to provide relief. Nephrostomy tubes may be needed.

Pulmonary Metastases

The lung is a common site of metastases. Metastases may present as solitary mass or multiple nodules. Eighty-five percent of pulmonary metastases are asymptomatic. Chest x-ray and CT scan are used for diagnosis. Resection of the metastatic area is the best option to achieve long-term survival, if possible. Prognosis is poor if resection is not possible.

Chapter 41
. . . .

Endocrine Cancers

THYROID TUMORS

Incidence

Thyroid tumors are rare, accounting for approximately 1% of total cancers and 0.2% of cancer deaths. Women have more than twice the risk of developing thyroid cancer. Most cases occur between ages 25 and 65.

Etiology

Individuals at increased risk for papillary thyroid cancer

- Individuals exposed to head and neck irradiation during childhood or adolescence
- Children who receive total body irradiation in preparation for allogeneic bone marrow transplant
- Individuals exposed to radiation from nuclear power plant disasters
- Benign thyroid disease
- Hormonal factors in women
- Diet deficient in iodine

Medullary thyroid cancer (MTC) is associated with genetically transmitted multiple endocrine neoplasia (MEN) syndrome.

Pathophysiology

Thyroid neoplasms include papillary, follicular, medullary, and anaplastic tumors.

Papillary Tumors

- Papillary tumors are multifocal and infiltrate local tissues.

PART VI

- Vascular invasion and metastasis to bone and lung occur.
- Women are three times more likely than men to develop papillary carcinomas.
- Papillary carcinomas are typically well-differentiated, indolent, and have a good prognosis.

Follicular Tumors
- Follicular thyroid cancer is more aggressive than papillary cancer.
- Follicular cancer is most often diagnosed in persons in their 50s.
- Hurthle cell carcinoma is a subtype of follicular carcinoma that occurs in older individuals and may cause hyperthyroidism.

Medullary Tumors
- Medullary thyroid tumors occur equally in men and women and constitute 5% to 10% of all thyroid carcinomas.
- 50% of patients will have tumor spread to their cervical lymph nodes.
- Ten-year survival is only 42% in patients with involved lymph nodes, and 90% in patients with negative regional lymph nodes.

Anaplastic Tumor
- 5% to 10% of thyroid malignancies are anaplastic.
- These tumors typically present as a fast-growing, invasive neck mass.
- Men and women in their 60s are at equal risk.
- Metastatic sites include lymph nodes, bone, and lung.

Clinical Manifestations
Manifestations are rarely present with early disease. An enlargement of the neck, neck pain, dysphagia, dysphonia, or hoarseness may cause an individual to seek medical care. MTC may present

as diarrhea secondary to hypersecretion of calcitonin.

Assessment

Diagnostic procedures for thyroid cancers

- History of exposure to radiation and family history, especially if familial MTC or MEN2 is suspected
- Physical examination may reveal a painless anterior cervical adenopathy or regional lymph
  node metastasis.
- A thyroid mass is usually found by the patient
  or on physical examination.
- Elevated serum calcitonin levels are suggestive
  of medullary hyperplasia or MTC.
- Ultrasonography or radionuclide scanning, CT,
  MRI, and PET scan all provide useful diagnostic
  information.
- Biopsy and histopathological examination of
  tumor tissue by fine-needle aspiration (FNA)
  confirms the diagnosis.

Treatment

Surgery

- Surgery is often reserved for the symptomatic
  patient. Risk of recurrence is 5% to 10% with
  lobectomy.
- When cure is possible, more aggressive surgery
  has been advocated for medullary and anaplastic tumors.
- Recurrent laryngeal nerve paralysis, vocal cord
  paralysis, thyroid storm, hemorrhage, and hypothyroidism are complications of surgery.
- The patient may require tracheostomy and gastrostomy, which can be performed at the time
  of initial surgery.
- If nodes are involved, lymph node dissection is
  indicated.

PART VI

- Thyroid suppressive treatment is given for several weeks before surgery to induce atrophy of the thyroid and reduce vascularity and hemorrhage at time of surgery.

PARATHYROID TUMORS

Incidence

Carcinomas account for less than 0.1% to 5.0% of primary hyperparathyroidism. Tumors occur equally in males and females. Parathyroid tumors most commonly occur in individuals who have familial MEN1, and less frequently in those with MEN2A. There are no significant risk factors for parathyroid carcinoma.

Pathophysiology

Local infiltration, invasion into blood vessels, and metastases characterize malignant tumors. Both benign and malignant parathyroid tumors are usually biochemically functional and hypersecrete (PTH), which leads to hypercalcemia. Twenty percent of patients have cervical lymph node metastases, and 16% have distant metastases, most commonly to the lungs, bone, or liver.

Clinical Manifestations

A palpable neck mass or hoarseness are manifestations of a parathyroid tumor. Symptoms of hypercalcemia include nausea, anorexia, weight loss, and dehydration.

Assessment

Diagnostic measures include nuclear scanning, CT, and ultrasound. FNA is not recommended because of the risk of tumor spread locally. When unexplained hypercalcemia is discovered, an immunoassay for immunoassayable parathyroid hormone is done. Approximately half of the patients with hyperparathyroidism have evidence of bony disease.

Treatment

Treatment includes surgery and chemotherapy. Surgery involves an en bloc resection of the abnormal parathyroid; if nodes are involved, radical neck dissection is done. Postoperative complications include hypoparathyroidism, recurrent laryngeal nerve damage, and hemorrhage.

Chemotherapy involves combination regimens, including 5-FU, cyclophosphamide, and dacarbazine or methotrexate, doxorubicin, and cyclophosphamide.

PITUITARY TUMORS

Incidence

Approximately 10% of brain tumors are pituitary tumors. Women are 4 times more likely than men to develop a prolactinoma. Seventy percent of pituitary adenomas occur in persons age 30 to 50, but these tumors also can develop in children.

Etiology

A pituitary tumor transforming gene has been cloned and is thought to play a role in tumorigenesis and progression. Genetic mutations in tumor-suppressor genes and oncogenes have been identified in pituitary tumors. Mutations in the *p53* gene are found in invasive pituitary adenomas and carcinomas.

Pathophysiology

The pituitary consists of the anterior and the posterior pituitary. The anterior pituitary controls growth by secreting trophic hormones (thyroid-stimulating hormone, adrenocorticotropin, prolactin, and growth hormone). Secretion of trophic hormones is regulated by negative-feedback loops that are influenced by the target organs.

Most pituitary tumors are localized, benign adenomas and are incapable of metastasizing. Adenomas grow by expansion to cause a mass effect. The tumors usually express altered gene products for neurotransmitters and hypothalamic hormones that cause physiological effects.

Clinical Manifestations

The signs and symptoms of pituitary adenomas result from secretion or depression of particular hormones or mass effect.

Hormone effects

- Prolactinomas
  - Prolactinomas constitute 60% of all functioning pituitary tumors.
  - Women are more likely to have small tumors that cause galactorrhea, menstrual irregularities, or infertility.
  - Men are more likely to have large tumors and high prolactin levels, with decreased libido or impotence.
- Growth hormone–secreting tumors
  - These tumors induce acromegaly in adults and gigantism in prepubescent children.
  - Early symptoms include fatigue or lethargy, paresthesia, and headache.
  - Other symptoms include weight gain, excessive perspiration, insulin resistance, and diabetes.
- Cushing's syndrome
  - Hypersecretion of ACTH by a pituitary adenoma is the major cause of Cushing's syndrome, resulting in 70% to 80% of all cases.
  - Symptoms include moon face, truncal obesity, hypertension, impaired glucose tolerance, and hypogonadism.
  - Congestive heart failure, purple striae, muscular weakness, pedal edema, skeletal pain, and psychological changes, and hirsutism in women.

Mass effects
- Headaches
- Visual changes
    - Diplopia due to compression of cranial nerves.
- Hypopituitarism due to tumor compression of the hypothalamus, pituitary stalk, or normal pituitary.
- Hormone insufficiency and altered secretion of posterior pituitary hormones, causing increased appetite, diabetes insipidus, or other effects

Assessment
Confirmation of a pituitary tumor includes the history and physical examination, endocrinology testing, radiological findings (CT and MRI), and histopathological examination.

Treatment
Surgery
Surgery is the treatment of choice for most pituitary tumors. The purpose of surgery is to resect or debulk large tumors compressing vital structures.

The surgical approach used most often is the transsphenoidal procedure, because the tumor can be removed and pituitary function can be preserved.

Radiation Therapy
Radiation therapy is used for patients who refuse or who cannot tolerate surgery, for tumor recurrence, or as an adjunct to surgery. Usual doses are 4500 to 5400 cGy given in 180- to 200-cGy daily fractions.

Drug Therapy
Drug therapy includes dopamine agonists and octreotide to treat hormone oversecretion.

ADRENAL TUMORS

Incidence

Adrenocortical tumors arise from the cortex, and pheochromocytomas arise from the medulla. Most are benign, but both adenomas and carcinomas may be life-threatening. Adrenocortical carcinomas are rare and occur in children under age 5 and in adults in their 40s and 50s. Pheochromocytomas are rare and arise from chromaffin cells. Both benign and malignant tumors synthesize, store, and release catecholamines and can lead to life-threatening myocardial infarction.

Etiology

Mutations of the *p53* gene have been documented in adults and children with adrenocortical carcinomas. Chronic stimulation of the adrenal cortex by pituitary hormones may initiate the random mutation. There are no known risk factors for adrenocortical tumors.

Pheochromocytomas occur sporadically and may be associated with hyperplasia. Increased expression of three genes for catecholamine synthesizing enzymes are present in tumor tissue.

Pathophysiology

Adrenocortical tumors may be functional (hormone-secreting) or nonfunctional (nonsecreting). Thirty percent to 50% hypersecrete cortisol to cause Cushing's syndrome; 20% to 30% secrete estradiol or testosterone to cause feminizing or masculinizing effects. Adrenocortical carcinomas are highly aggressive, and 50% to 70% of patients have locally advanced disease at presentation.

Pheochromocytomas hypersecrete the catecholamine norepinephrine. After the initial diagnosis, they may recur in the surgical bed or at distant sites in lymph nodes, bone, lung, liver, and brain.

Clinical Manifestations

The signs and symptoms of adrenocortical tumors vary, depending on the hormone secreted or the symptoms from local mass effects. Patients with nonfunctional tumors usually have a palpable abdominal mass and may have abdominal or back pain. Fever, weight loss, weakness, and lethargy are seen primarily in patients with advanced disease.

Patients with aldosterone-hypersecreting tumors present with hypertension, hypokalemia, and hypernatremia. Most functional tumors result in Cushing's disease and virilization and feminization syndromes.

Pheochromocytomas producing catecholamines present with headache, palpitations, sweating, anxiety, nausea, and vomiting.

Assessment

Functional adrenocortical tumors are detected by immunoassays of hormone precursors and urinary excretion tests, because hormone metabolites are excreted in the urine. Localization or imaging procedures to examine the adrenal cortex may include CT or MRI.

Urinary secretion tests for circulating catecholamines or their metabolites are the most sensitive in detecting pheochromocytoma. CT and MRI scans are used to localize the tumor.

Treatment

Surgery is the treatment of choice for adrenocortical tumors and may be curative for localized disease. Glucocorticoid treatment may be needed either temporarily or permanently. Almost 80% of patients develop recurrent regional disease or distant metastasis. Mitotane may be given with surgery to control hormone hypersecretion in cortical tumors.

Pheochromocytomas are also curable by surgery; however, the patient is monitored carefully for uncontrolled hypertension. Patients are often

PART VI

placed on alpha-adrenergic medications to decrease the risk of crisis during surgery and postoperative hypotension. Radiation and chemotherapy have little effect in pheochromocytomas and, in fact, may trigger severe hypertension due to rapid cellular release of norepinephrine following tumor lysis.

MULTIPLE ENDOCRINE NEOPLASIA (MEN SYNDROME)

MEN syndromes are almost always caused by an inherited gene mutation in which several endocrine malignancies occur. Manifestations of MEN vary, depending on which organs are involved and whether tumors secrete hormones.

Screening for affected individuals in families known to express MEN is the major focus of management. Genetic testing in family members with a known risk for MEN is the diagnostic method of choice. Treatment involves surgery of the affected gland and can involve multiple glands.

Chapter 42

Endometrial Cancers

Incidence

Endometrial cancer is the predominant cancer of the female genital tract. About 38,300 new cases are predicted for 2001. Fortunately, the mortality rate is low. Approximately 6600 women are predicted to die of the disease in 2001.

Endometrial cancer is primarily a disease of post-menopausal women. It commonly occurs in women between ages 50 and 59. In most cases, the diagnosis is made when disease is localized.

Overall survival rates:

- Stage I: 76%
- Stage II: 50%
- Stage III: 30%
- Stage IV: 9%

Etiology

Risk Factors

- Obesity (more than 20 lb. overweight)
- Diabetes
- Hypertension
- Reproductive factors
  - Nulliparity
  - Late menopause (after age 52)
  - Infertility
  - Irregular menses
  - Failure of ovulation
- History of colorectal, breast, or ovarian cancer
- Tamoxifen use
- Estrogen replacement without adequate progesterone

PART VI

A healthy lifestyle of a low-fat diet, regular physical activity, and maintaining normal weight may contribute to risk reduction. Two factors appear to have a protective effect against the development of endometrial cancer:

1. Oral contraceptives
2. Smoking (risk of lung cancer and other problems far outweighs protection)

Pathophysiology

Most endometrial cancers are adenocarcinomas. Cancer usually starts in the fundus and may spread to involve the entire endometrium. Metastatic spread is usually by direct extension and pelvic and paraaortic nodes. Other sites of spread are lung, liver, bone, and brain.

Multiple factors affect the natural history and prognosis of endometrial cancer (Table 42.1).

Clinical Manifestations

The hallmark signal of endometrial cancer is abnormal or new vaginal bleeding. Postmenopausal bleeding is another warning sign that should be investigated immediately. Less common symptoms are premenopausal onset of heavy or irregular bleeding, pyometra, hematuria, and lumbosacral, hypogastric, or pelvic pain.

Table 42.1 Prognostic Indicators

Indicator	Good Prognosis	Poor Prognosis
Stage of disease	I	II, III, IV
Histology	Adenocarcinomas; non-serous, non-clear cell	Serous or clear cell
Tumor differentiation	Grade I	Grades 2, 3
Myometrial invasion	Superficial or none	Deep (>50%)
Nodal metastasis	None	Present
Peritoneal cytology	Negative	Positive

Assessment

Patient and Family History
A thorough history should include evaluation of potential risk factors, and focus on

- description of presenting symptoms,
- reproductive history,
- estrogen use,
- tamoxifen use, and
- dietary habits.

Physical Examination
- Nodal surveillance
- Palpation of abdomen for evidence of disease
- Complete pelvic examination

Diagnostic Measures
A Pap smear occasionally detects an endometrial cancer.

More reliable diagnostic techniques

- Endometrial biopsy (90% effective in detection)
- If biopsy is negative and symptoms persist, D&C
- Chest x-ray
- Hematological profiles
- Cystoscopy, barium enema, proctoscopy

Classification and Staging
Endometrial cancer is staged surgically according to the Corpus Cancer Staging by the International Federation of Gynecology and Obstetrics. Surgical staging procedures involve

- bimanual examination,
- peritoneal cytology,
- inspection and palpation of peritoneal surfaces,
- biopsies, and
- selective pelvic and paraaortic lymphadenectomy.

PART VI

Treatment
Definitive treatment depends on the stage of the disease.

Early Stage Disease (Stages I and II)
The goal of treatment is cure and long-term survival. Early disease is usually treated as follows:

- Surgery
  - Total abdominal hysterectomy, bilateral salpingo-oophorectomy, selective lymphadenectomy, omentectomy, and peritoneal washings
- Radiation therapy
  - If there is positive peritoneal cytology, intraperitoneal radioactive colloidal phosphorus can be helpful. External beam therapy is used for disease localized to the pelvis. Whole-pelvis radiation allows treatment of all pelvic tissue.

Advanced or Recurrent Disease (Stage III or IV)
The goal of treatment is to control the disease and the associated symptoms. Long-term survival is rare. Treatment includes the following:

- Surgery and radiation
  - Vaginal recurrences confined to the vagina are treated with surgery or radiotherapy. Recurrences outside the vagina require multimodal therapy.
- Hormonal therapy
  - Synthetic progestational agents (e.g., megestrol acetate and medroxyprogesterone) produce 30% to 37% response rates. Receptor status greatly affects response. If both estrogen and progesterone receptors are positive, the response rate is about 77%. If not, response is poor. Side effects of hormone therapy include fluid retention, phlebitis, and thrombosis.

- Chemotherapy
  - Few cytotoxic agents have demonstrated activity greater than hormone therapy. Combination chemotherapy using doxorubicin and cisplatin is used predominantly.

Supportive Care

The woman with early-stage endometrial cancer can expect long-term disease-free survival. Health maintenance is a major part of ongoing care. Information needs and supportive care following treatment for endometrial cancer include the following:

- Estrogen replacement therapy (ERT) is indicated for most women because their ovaries have been removed or ablated during definitive therapy. ERT is often prescribed if the woman experiences
  - vaginal atrophy, with infection or sexual dysfunction;
  - loss of pelvic support, with incontinence;
  - postmenopausal osteoporosis;
  - perimenopausal emotional lability; or
  - vasomotor instability.
- Annual pelvic examinations, breast self-examination, diet and weight control, and exercise are excellent preventive measures to teach and reinforce with the woman following therapy for endometrial cancer.
- Abnormal vaginal bleeding is a sign that requires immediate attention. Usually, a pelvic examination and laparoscopy will be done to determine whether there is recurrence.
- Psychosexual concerns need to be discussed because many women fear the loss of femininity due to removal of the uterus or ovaries. A complete sexual assessment may be indicated if the woman is anxious. Review the anatomic alterations and potential side effects of therapy along with suggestions for management:

- Alteration in sexual response can occur secondary to hysterectomy. The cervix contributes to, but is not essential for, orgasm. The uterus elevates during the excitement phase and contracts rhythmically during orgasm. Prepare the woman to anticipate that orgasms can still be achieved.

- Alteration in sexual functioning can occur secondary to radiation. Vaginal dryness and stenosis may result in the patient who is not sexually active, unless vaginal dilators and lubricants are employed. Encourage the woman to use water-soluble lubricants during intercourse and to use nonhormonal moisturizers three times per week to help with the dryness.

The woman with advanced end-stage endometrial cancer may experience pelvic pain from tumor invasion; hematuria, if the bladder is involved; fecal incontinence, if a rectovaginal fistula develops; obstruction of the bowel; or lung metastases. Each of these challenges is handled with aggressive palliative approaches.

Chapter 43
....

Esophageal Cancer

Incidence
Esophageal cancer is uncommon in the United States. It represents less than 1% of all cancer cases. There are about 12,000 new cases diagnosed each year. It is more common among men than women. The highest incidence occurs after age 50.

Squamous cell carcinoma is more common among Asians and African Americans. Adenocarcinoma is more common among Whites.

Etiology
The esophagus is subject to many factors that can affect the health of the tissues, such as type and temperature of food, acid reflux from the stomach, and overflow of substances inhaled into the trachea. The cause of esophageal cancer is not completely known, but it is probably multifaceted.

Risk Factors
- Heavy alcohol intake
- Heavy tobacco use
- Barrett's esophagus
- Poor nutrition
- High nitrosamine intake in food
- Viral infection (human papilloma virus)
- Mutations of tumor-suppressor genes *p53* and APC

Pathophysiology

Cellular Characteristics
There are two main histological types of esophageal cancer:

1. Squamous cell carcinoma: predominant cell type, usually better differentiated, more common in proximal and mid-esophagus
2. Adenocarcinoma: typically arises in distal esophagus

Progression of Disease

Esophageal tumors grow rapidly, metastasize early, and are usually diagnosed late. Progression of the disease occurs by direct extension, especially early in the disease. Later, the tumors progress into the regional lymph nodes. The most common sites of metastases are the left mainstem bronchus, thoracic duct, aortic arch, pleura, pericardium, and diaphragm.

Prognostic Indicators

The prognosis for esophageal cancer is poor. Two key prognostic indicators are the depth of tumor invasion and presence of abdominal metastases. Patients with T3N0 have a 50% chance of living 5 years.

Clinical Manifestations

Many people mistakenly attribute signs and symptoms of esophageal cancer to disorders of digestion that commonly affect older persons. The early symptoms may be nonspecific and of little concern. Dysphagia and weight loss are the most common presenting symptoms. Dysphagia is progressive and pain on swallowing, loss of appetite, and malaise may also be present.

Assessment

Physical examination is not particularly helpful. Endoscopy with biopsy is the only definitive method for diagnosis. Endoscopic ultrasound and CT scan are used for staging. Routine x-ray films and double-barium contrast studies, and positron emission tomography (PET) can be used to further define the tumor.

Classification and Staging

Classification is based on the TNM system. Staging involves both clinical and pathological staging. The majority of people with esophageal cancer present with T3N1 or T4 disease.

Treatment

Treatment approaches to esophageal cancer are varied and depend on the stage of the disease and the general health of the patient. Tumor invasion of the bronchus usually makes the tumor unresectable. In addition, the presence of metastases eliminates surgery as a treatment option in most cases. The treatment approach is different for the extent of disease and various anatomical sites within the esophagus, as follows.

Local and Locoregional Esophageal Cancer

Surgery

Surgery is used as the primary treatment for those with resectable disease that is considered local or locoregional. Depending on the location of the tumor, surgical approaches for local disease include the following:

- Radical esophagectomy to remove the entire esophagus; associated with high mortality rate
- Abdominal and right thoracotomy for cancers of the upper and middle third of the esophagus. This procedure allows good visualization of the involved area.
- Left transthoracic approach for cancers of the lower third of the esophagus, which involves an incision across the abdomen and thorax
- Transhiatal esophagectomy for cancer at all three levels. This has been performed more extensively in recent years because it avoids a thoracotomy and its complications.
- Reconstruction of esophageal continuity can be achieved by elevating the stomach to create esophagogastrectomy, interposing a segment of

PART VI

the colon, and elevating the gastric tube created from the stomach to reconstruct a lumen.

Potential postoperative complications of esophageal cancer surgeries

- Fistula
- Anastomotic leak
- Atelectasis
- Pneumonia
- Pulmonary edema
- Cardiac problems

Important nursing measures to anticipate and to manage the preceding postoperative complications

- Aggressive respiratory care
- Chest physiotherapy
- Tracheobronchial hygiene
- Prevention of fluid overload
- Prevention of infection
- Meticulous suture line care
- Monitoring of drainage, output
- Maintenance of patent gastrointestinal tubes
- Helping patient maintain body alignment
- Detection of fistulas
- Prevention of reflux aspiration
- Elevation of head of bed
- Encouraging patient not to consume snacks or liquid after evening meal
- Encouraging patient to eat small amounts of food more often
- Encouraging patient to avoid bending from waist
- Encouraging patient to avoid heavy lifting

Combined Therapy

Surgery, radiation, and chemotherapy are options to treat local and locoregional disease. Combination therapy offers the best alternative for resectable disease. Cisplatin and 5-FU are the chemotherapy agents most commonly used. Radiation doses of 2000 cGy to 4500 cGy are typical for combination therapy plans.

Combined therapy approaches result in greater toxicities of myelosuppression, neutropenia, nutritional disturbances, fatigue, and drug-specific side effects. The side effects can be managed and treatment continued.

Nonresectable or Metastatic Disease

Nonresectable or metastatic disease requires aggressive palliative therapy to prevent the debilitating effects of obstruction of the major entryway to the intestinal tract. Nonresectable esophageal tumors are often treated as follows:

- Radiotherapy alone or in combination with chemotherapy
- Brachytherapy alone or in combination with external beam therapy
- Esophageal dilatation can temporarily alleviate dysphagia
- An esophageal stent can be placed to provide a more lasting opening of the esophagus.
- Laser therapy and photodynamic therapy are options used to shrink and palliate accessible tumors causing either partial or total obstruction of the passage.

Supportive Care

The objective of supportive care is to relieve the distressing symptoms caused by advanced esophageal cancer. Progressive dysphagia and weight loss are the most debilitating symptoms. Tube feedings may be necessary to sustain nutrition. Patients with obstruction of the esophagus may have trouble clearing secretions, and sleeping with the bed elevated can help prevent a feeling of choking.

Hemorrhage may occur if the esophageal tumor erodes surrounding tissues, requiring emergency surgery. Hepatic failure can result from liver metastases. Pain associated with bone metastases requires aggressive pain control.

Chapter 44

Gallbladder Cancer

Incidence
Gallbladder cancer is rare, with only about 6000 cases diagnosed each year. Incidence is highest in southwest regions of the United States among Native Americans and Hispanic Americans. Women develop gallbladder cancer twice as often as men, and incidence is highest after age 50.

Etiology
Several factors are associated with an increased risk for gallbladder cancer.

- Gallstones (single gallstone, usually larger than 3 cm)
- Gallbladder polyps
- Calcification of the gallbladder wall
- Choledochal cyst
- Anomalous pancreatobiliary duct junction
- Obesity
- Carcinogens (rubber plant workers, azotoluene, nitrosamines)
- Estrogens
- Typhoid carriers

Pathophysiology
The majority of tumors (85%) are adenocarcinomas. Gallbladder cancer invades locally into the liver, duodenum, transverse colon, portal vein, or pancreas. Biliary obstruction is a common sequela.

PART VI

Clinical Manifestations
Gallbladder cancer is usually asymptomatic in the early stages, which precludes early diagnosis.

When symptomatic, common symptoms are

- right upper abdominal pain,
- nausea and vomiting,
- fatty-food intolerance, and
- chills and fever.

Nonspecific symptoms associated with advanced disease include

- malaise,
- anorexia,
- weight loss,
- abdominal distention,
- pruritus, and
- jaundice.

Assessment

Physical examination may reveal a distended gallbladder when the patient is supine. Diagnostic studies are not usually definitive. Ultrasound, CT, MRI, cholangiography, and angiography may help diagnosis.

Histological grade has significant prognostic implications. Metaplasia correlates with a poor prognosis. Degree of invasion by the tumor is predictive of survival.

Classification and Staging

The TNM staging system is commonly used. Histological grading on the basis of differentiation and the degree of invasion are important factors in staging.

Treatment

The stage of the tumor and degree of invasion influence the choice of treatment. Liver problems such as cirrhosis may increase surgical risk.

Surgery

The most effective treatment is surgical resection, but fewer than 25% of gallbladder cancers are resectable. Cholecystectomy is the primary treatment for stage I tumors. If the tumor is limited to the mucosa, simple cholecystectomy is best. Laparoscopic removal is not recommended because it may lead to tumor dissemination in the abdomen. If tumor involves deeper layers of the gallbladder wall, radical or extended cholecystectomy can be performed, despite a grim prognosis.

Local invasion of the liver can be handled with a wedge resection, but more extensive involvement of the liver may necessitate a larger resection.

Radiation Therapy and Chemotherapy
Radiation can be used for both resectable and nonresectable disease. No survival advantage has been noted. Chemotherapy agents have been limited due to poor tumor response.

Palliative Therapy
Many people with gallbladder cancer have obstructive jaundice, which can be relieved with an endoscopically placed stent or prosthesis. Pain relief, radiation, gastrojejunostomy bypass, and antisecretory agents may be used. Most patients with unresectable disease do not survive more than 4 months.

Chapter 45

Head and Neck Malignancies

Incidence

Head and neck cancer accounts for a small percentage of newly diagnosed cancers in the United States (males, 5%; females, 2%). Incidence rates for men are twice as high as for women. Black men have the overall highest incidence of oral cavity cancer. The fifth most frequent cause of cancer death in the Alaska native population among males is nasopharyngeal cancer.

Etiology

Tobacco abuse has been implicated for all head and neck tumor sites.

Risk Factors

- Use of tobacco, including cigarettes, smokeless tobacco, pipes, cigars, and marijuana
- Use of alcohol; there also may be synergism between alcohol and tobacco
- Exposure to dust from wood, metal, leather, textiles, or chemical inhalants
- Poor oral hygiene; chronic irritation from loose-fitting dentures
- Epstein-Barr virus (EBV) and nasopharyngeal cancer
- Genetic predisposition
- Nutritional deficiencies, such as Plummer-Vinson syndrome
- Vitamin A deficiency

Pathophysiology

Most cancers of the head and neck originate in the epithelial tissue and are classifed as squamous cell carcinomas (SCCs). The other tumor type is adenocarcinoma, which originates from the major or minor salivary glands. Head and neck tumors are graded as either well-, moderately-, or poorly differentiated tumors. Prognosis for cure correlates with the degree of loss of differentiation. The incidence of spread to regional lymph nodes at diagnosis is high. These tumors tend to recur locally, and when there is involvement of distant lymph nodes, the cancer is classified as metastatic.

Clinical Manifestations

Table 45.1 lists symptoms of the various head and neck cancers. Common symptoms for all sites include weight loss and a persistent lump or mass, unilaterally.

Table 45.1 Symptoms of Head and Neck Cancers	
Tumor Site	**Symptoms**
Oral cavity (lip, floor of mouth, tongue, hard palate)	Loosening teeth or ill-fitting dentures, swelling of gums, dysplasia, hyperplasia, pain, nonhealing lesion, bleeding
Nose and paranasal sinuses	Unilateral obstruction of naris, nonhealing ulcer, intermittent epistaxis
Nasopharynx	Nasal obstruction, pain, otological changes
Oropharynx (base of tongue, tonsil, soft palate)	Asymmetry, dull ache, pain, dysphagia, erythroplakia, otalgia, trismus
Larynx and hypopharynx	
Supraglottic	Dysphagia, odynophagias, aspiration, referred otalgia, tickling sensation in throat
Glottic	Throat irritation, dysphagia, hoarseness, dyspnea, and stridor with large tumors
Subglottic	Dyspnea, stridor, and hemoptysis
Salivary gland	Unilateral symptoms, impaired jaw mobility, numb lower lip

Assessment

Because the initial symptoms may be silent, the person with a head and neck tumor may present with significant malignant changes, even though regular physical examinations have taken place. In addition to a complete physical examination, a complete nutritional assessment helps with future nutritional interventions.

Diagnostic Measures

Various tests may be necessary for diagnosis and determining treatment.

- Nasopharyngoscopy with biopsies
- Direct laryngoscopy
- Plain x-ray films
- CT scan or MRI
- Angiography

Classification and Staging

Classification and staging of head and neck cancers is specific to each primary site. The American Joint Committee on Cancer TNM staging system is used.

Treatment

Treatment is according to the anatomical location of the tumor. Early disease may be treated with either radiation or surgery; more advanced disease is usually treated with a combination of radiation, surgery, and, sometimes, chemotherapy.

Nasal Fossa and Paranasal Sinuses

- Maxillectomy is the treatment of choice for tumors in the maxillary sinus; a combination of radical maxillectomy and orbital exenteration may be performed if there is extensive disease with invasion into the floor of the orbit.
- An obturator is made and placed at the time of surgery to restore nasal continuity, allow the patient to eat and speak immediately after surgery, and protect the wound from irritation and

debris. The obturator remains in place for 5 days; it is then removed and replaced with a more permanent obturator.

- The patient is taught to remove the obturator after each meal, irrigate it with alkaline-based fluid, and remove any crusting-over defect. The obturator is not removed for long periods of time, as atrophy can occur.

Carcinoma of the Skull Base
- Surgery is used to resect tumors that involve or have extended to the skull base.
- Complications can include cerebral edema thrombosis, seizures, stroke, and infections.

Carcinoma of the Nasopharynx
- High-dose, external beam radiation therapy is used.
- Surgery is not usually recommended due to difficult access to this site.
- For local, recurrent disease, brachytherapy alone or in conjunction with radiation therapy may be the best approach.
- Chemotherapy is often given in conjunction with radiation therapy for advanced disease.

Carcinoma of the Oral Cavity
- In early-stage lesions, surgery or radiation alone have comparable cure rates; choice of treatment depends on the functional and cosmetic results required, the patient's general health, and the patient's preference.
- Laser therapy may better preserve function for patients with early-stage, transoral resections.
- Advanced tumors are usually managed with a combination of surgery and radiation therapy.
- With oral cavity tumors, surgical resection often involves neck dissection, depending on stage and regional spread, followed by radiation therapy.

- Speaking and swallowing can be greatly affected, depending on location of tumor.

Carcinoma of the Oropharynx

- In early-stage lesions, surgery or radiation alone have comparable cure rates; choice of treatment depends on the functional and cosmetic results required.
- Tonsil malignancies are treated with radiation therapy.
- High-dose irradiation, often with brachytherapy may be used for posterior tumors of the tongue because of severe functional impairment.
- For advanced posterior tongue tumors, treatment is usually a total laryngectomy in conjunction with total resection of the tongue base.

Carcinoma of the Salivary Gland

- Parotid tumors require a superficial parotidectomy with facial nerve dissection.
- Adjuvant radiation therapy is generally given to all postoperative patients.

Carcinoma of Larynx

Supraglottic Carcinoma

- Early-stage disease is treated by either partial laryngectomy or radiation therapy.
- Due to the likelihood of cervical spread, a neck dissection is selected according to nodal involvement.

Glottic Carcinomas

- Unlike supraglottic tumors, glottic cancers initially remain localized, and lymphatic spread is limited.
- In situ tumors may be treated with laser vaporization, microexcision, or radiation therapy.
- In advanced cases, patients are treated with either a total laryngectomy plus neck dissection and adjuvant radiation therapy or radiation

therapy followed by surgical salvage, as necessary, for persistent disease.

- With total laryngectomy plus neck dissection, as well as permanent voice loss and alternation of airway, fistula formation, carotid rupture, wound infections, and pharyngeal stenosis can occur as postoperative complications.

- Organ (larynx) preservation protocols with chemoradiation are becoming more widely used.

Carcinoma of the Hypopharynx

- Radiation therapy is frequently recommended for individuals with early-stage disease in order to preserve the voice.

- In the event of recurrence, a total laryngectomy is usually done.

- Chemotherapy may be used preoperatively to shrink the tumor to operable status.

Surgical Restoration: Reconstruction and Rehabilitation

Prior to surgery, the surgeon will anticipate the location and dimensions of the surgical defect. The goal is to restore function and maintain socially adequate cosmesis by covering the surgical defect by a flap or graft following tumor removal.

- Local skin flaps are used to cover areas with partial- to full-thickness loss and organized according to the vascular supply of the site.

- Free flaps can be customized and harvested according to the needs and size of the defect.

- Full-thickness and split-thickness skin grafts are secured by suturing the graft into the recipient defect.

- Full-thickness grafts are usually harvested from areas of the body that have natural creases (e.g., preauricular).

- Split-thickness grafts are nearly transparent and are usually taken from the lateral thigh.

PART VI

Supportive Care

Airway Management

Tracheostomy and laryngectomy care

- If tumor affects the patient's breathing or if surgical procedure includes the compromised airway, a tracheostomy is necessary.
- At the time of surgery, a cuffed tracheostomy tube is usually sutured in place, and patients are taught how to suction the tracheostomy tube, remove and clean inner cannula, clean the tracheostoma, and apply a clean dressing, as necessary.
- The tracheostomy or laryngectomy tube is removed when it is no longer needed; the slit incision is taped, and the site heals over in 4 to 6 weeks.
- Adequate humidity is crucial, because individuals with altered airways have lost the ability of the nose to moisten, warm, or filter the air they breathe. Supplemental humidity is necessary.
- Teach patients the importance of mobilizing secretions by coughing, drinking adequate fluids, and instilling saline into the stoma to loosen secretions, if necessary.

Nutritional Support

- Ongoing consultation with the nutritionist is important throughout treatment.
- If the patient has trouble swallowing, tube feedings will become necessary.

Swallowing Rehabilitation

- Preservation and/or restoration of the swallowing function is a primary rehabilitation goal.
- When the physiology of the oral cavity has been compromised (e.g., resection of the tongue, nerve damage), the patient will need to learn methods to propel foods for swallowing.

Speech Restoration

- Restorative speech methods for total laryngectomy patients

  - Artificial larynx: an electronic, vibrating device that resonates sound into the oral cavity; easy to learn how to use.

  - Esophageal speech: Swallowing air into the esophagus, the person articulates instantly with the expulsion of air to form speech. No equipment is required. It may take up to 6 months to learn this technique.

  - Tracheoesophageal puncture (TEP): one-way plastic valve prosthesis that fits into tracheoesophageal slit. Provides for airflow from the lung to the esophagus to the mouth when the stoma is occluded and results in easy-to-learn speech. The patient must learn to clean, maintain, and insert the prosthesis.

Psychosocial Support

- Head and neck malignancies are devastating. Key senses, such as sight, taste, smell, hearing, and touch, may be permanently impaired.

- Disfiguring surgery has a major impact on self- and body image.

- It is important to be supportive and partner with the patient during the evolution of the treatment process.

Chapter 46

Hodgkin's Disease

Incidence
Hodgkin's disease (HD) accounts for 11% of the malignant lymphomas and less than 1% of all cancers. The incidence of HD has two peaks:

1. Young adults aged 20 to 30
2. Adults over age 45 (HD increases steadily to the seventh and eighth decades)

Histological category and anatomical distribution also vary by age.

Etiology
The etiology of HD remains unclear. An infectious source has been speculated and the role of viruses, especially the Epstein-Barr virus (EBV), remains an important consideration. Genetic predispositions for HD also may exist.

Pathophysiology
HD is distinguished from other lymphomas by the presence of the Reed-Sternberg cell. HD patients exhibit a molecular defect characterized by markedly reduced cellular immunity and manifested by hypersensitivity skin reactions and reduced T-cell proliferation. They also display increased susceptibility to infections. The spread of HD is via contiguous nodal groups.

Clinical Manifestations
The HD patient typically presents with the following signs and symptoms:

- Enlarged lymph nodes (> 1 cm)
  - Painless, rubbery, and moveable
  - Most located in the cervical and supraclavicular areas

- Axillary and inguinal involvement in fewer than 10% of patients
- Mediastinal adenopathy is common.
- Constitutional symptoms, or "B" symptoms, are more common in advanced disease and include
  - fever,
  - nightsweats,
  - weight loss (> 10% of normal body weight),
  - malaise, and
  - pruritus (40% of patients).

Assessment

The diagnosis of HD can be established only by biopsy of the involved tissue, usually a lymph node. Occasionally, multiple biopsies are necessary for proper evaluation. In addition to a careful history and physical examination and routine laboratory work, the following diagnostic procedures are used for staging evaluation:

- Surgical lymph node biopsy
- Chest and abdominal CT and MRI
- Bipedal lymphangiogram if HD presents with inguinal or femoral nodal involvement
- Bilateral needle biopsy of iliac crests
- Evaluation of suspected extranodal disease

Classification and Staging

Once a diagnosis is confirmed, it is necessary to obtain accurate histological typing and staging of the disease in order to determine the precise prognosis and selection of therapy. There are five distinct subtypes of HD, and each category has well-defined characteristics and certain features (Table 46.1).

Treatment

The majority of patients are potentially curable if optimal therapy is used. Treatment success depends on the dosage and timing of drug adminis-

PART VI

Table 46.1	Classification of Hodgkin's Disease	
Histology	Frequency (%)	Features
Nodular sclerosis	60–80	Adolescents and young adults usually stage I or II; females predominate
Nodular lymphocyte-predominant	6–9	Adults in 30s usually stage I or II; males predominate; good prognosis
Diffuse lymphocyte-predominant	3–6	Presentation and survival are like mixed cellularity
Mixed cellularity	15–30	Males predominate; B symptoms common; majority have stage III or IV; intermediate prognosis
Lymphocyte-depleted	< 1	Older males predominate; B symptoms; widespread dissemination; poor prognosis

The Ann Arbor Cotswold staging system is used for HD.

tration, because even minor alterations can impact efficacy.

Guidelines for treatment of HD

- Radiation therapy for early-stage disease (stages I and II)
- Chemotherapy for early-stage and advanced-stage disease
- Radiation therapy and combination chemotherapy for patients with mediastinal disease, B symptoms, and abdominal nodes
- Combination chemotherapy involves the following drugs:
  - Mechlorethamine, vincristine, procarbazine, and prednisone (MOPP regimen)
  - Doxorubicin, bleomycin, vinblastine, and dacarbazine (ABVD regimen)
- If the patient relapses more than 12 months after initial therapy, the patient may be treated with the same agents.

- If the patient relapses less than 12 months after initial therapy, prognosis is poor.

Long-term complications in cured patients

- Gonadal dysfunction
- Second malignancies
- Progressive radiation myelopathy
- Pneumonitis
- Herpes zoster
- Pericarditis and cardiomyopathy

Supportive Care

Nurses play a pivotal role in promoting compliance with the treatment protocol by providing emotional support, effective symptom management, and reassurance about the treatment program. Reproductive counseling and sperm banking should be considered for the young patient.

Chapter 47

Kidney Cancer

Incidence

The two major types of kidney cancer are renal cell cancer and cancer of the renal pelvis. Renal cell cancer is more common, accounting for 3% of all cancers and 85% of all kidney cancers.

The four major variables related to incidence of kidney cancer:

1. Race: equivalent between whites and blacks but one-third greater in Hispanics than in Whites
2. Gender: 2 : 1 male predominance in renal cell cancer
3. Age: occurs most often between 50 and 70 years of age
4. Geographic: high incidence in Scandinavian countries, low in Japan, and intermediate in the United States

Etiology

Risk Factors

- Smoking (cigarette, cigar, pipe)
- Occupational exposure to hydrocarbon, cadmium, asbestos, and lead
- Heavy use of analgesics (e.g., aspirin, phenacetin, acetaminophen)
- Genetic factors (renal cell carcinoma)

Pathophysiology

Cellular Characteristics

Histologically, renal cell tumors are clear-cell, glandular-cell, or mixed-cell tumors. Tumors usually arise as a solitary, unilateral mass. The size of the tumor varies from a few centimeters to large tumors filling the peritoneal space.

Tumors of the renal pelvis arise from the epithelial tissue anywhere in the renal pelvis. These tumors often have independent, multifocal origins. The majority of renal pelvis cell types are transitional cell or squamous cell.

Progression of Disease
Renal cell tumors can be localized, spread by direct extension to the renal vein and into the vena cava or perinephric fat, or spread through the vasculature or lymphatics to distant sites. The most common sites of metastatic spread are the lungs, bone, lymph nodes, and brain.

Renal pelvis tumors may extend into the ureter and through the muscular coats.

Prognostic Indicators
Survival rates for renal cell cancer depend on the stage of disease. For patients with tumor confined to the kidney, the 5-year survival rate is 89%. The 5-year survival rate for all stages of kidney cancer is 61%.

Clinical Manifestations
The most common signs and symptoms for kidney cancers

- Hematuria (50%–60% of patients)
- Pain (40% of patients)
- Palpable flank or abdominal mass (30%–40% of patients)
- Fever
- Weight loss
- Anemia
- High association with paraneoplastic syndromes
- 30% to 50% of patients have metastasis at diagnosis.

Assessment

The most useful tests for renal cell carcinoma

- Computerized tomography
- Magnetic resonance imaging
- DNA flow cytometry
- Excretory urogram (intravenous pyelogram)
- Ultrasound
- Renal arteriography

The most useful tests to diagnose cancer of the renal pelvis

- Excretory urogram
- Retrograde urogram
- Urinary cytology
- CT, MRI, ultrasound

Classification and Staging

The TNM staging system and the Robson staging system are used for renal cell carcinoma. The TNM staging system is used for cancer of the renal pelvis.

Treatment

Renal Cell Carcinoma

- Radical nephrectomy
- Regional lymphadenectomy (controversial)
- Radiation therapy: effective palliation for metastatic disease
- Chemotherapy: no demonstrated response in renal cell carcinoma
- Interleukin-2 and interferon therapy: favorable response rates

Renal Pelvis Cancers

- Nephroureterectomy
- Percutaneous or ureteroscopic resection, followed by laser irradiation or intracavitary BCG or epidoxorubicin

Supportive Care

Preoperative and postoperative nursing care of the patient undergoing radical nephrectomy is similar to that of the individual undergoing laparotomy or pelvic surgery. The patient should be taught to report any symptoms of respiratory distress, pain, hemoptysis, or fracture, as these symptoms may signify metastasis. The importance of follow-up care and examinations should be stressed.

Chapter 48

Leukemias

Incidence

The leukemias represent a group of hematological malignancies that affect bone marrow and lymphatic tissue. Approximately half of the cases are acute and others are chronic. The number of new cases each year is greater in adults than in children.

The most common types of leukemia

- Acute myelogenous leukemia (AML)
  - Median age at diagnosis: 50 to 60 years
- Acute lymphocytic leukemia (ALL)
  - More common in children
- Chronic myelogenous leukemia (CML)
  - Peak incidence: third and fourth decades
  - Both sexes affected
- Chronic lymphocytic leukemia (CLL)
  - Median age at diagnosis: 70 years
  - More common in males

Etiology

The cause of leukemia is not known, but the following are the commonly considered etiological factors:

- Genetic factors
  - Family clustering
  - Chromosomal abnormalities
- Radiation
- Chemical exposure
  - Benzene
  - Paint
  - Dye

- Drugs
  - Alkylating agents
  - Chloramphenicol
  - Phenylbutazone
- Viruses

Pathophysiology

The regulatory mechanisms that control cell numbers and growth are missing or abnormal, which results in the following:

- Arrest of the cell in an early phase of its maturation process, causing an accumulation of immature cells
- An abnormal proliferation of these immature cells
- Crowding of other marrow elements, resulting in eventual replacement of the marrow by leukemic cells.

Leukemias are classified as either chronic or acute and as either myeloid or lymphoid. The type of leukemia is named according to the point at which cell maturation is arrested. In chronic leukemia, the cell is mature but does not function normally. In acute leukemia, the cell is immature.

Clinical Manifestations

Manifestations of leukemia are related to three factors:

1. An increase in immature white cells in bone marrow, spleen, liver, and lymph nodes
2. Infiltration of these leukemic cells into body tissues
3. A decrease in leukocytes, thrombocytes, and erythrocytes resulting from crowding of bone marrow with leukemic cells

However, these manifestations vary with each type of leukemia. The assessment and treatment for each major type are discussed separately.

PART VI

ACUTE LEUKEMIA

Assessment

Patient History and Physical Examination

The most common complaints of the patient are nonspecific (e.g., fever, weight loss, fatigue, sore throat). Other complaints and presenting symptoms:

- Recurrent infections
- Unexplained bleeding (e.g., bruising, petechiae, nosebleeds)
- Progressive anemia, with shortness of breath, splenomegaly, weakness, and fatigue
- Joint pain
- Neurological complaints (e.g., headache, vomiting, visual disturbances)

A comprehensive physical examination validates findings elicited in a complete history and review of symptoms.

Diagnostic Measures

It is important to differentiate between AML and ALL, because treatment and prognosis are very different. The diagnosis is suggested by the peripheral smear, but requires the following:

- Bone marrow biopsy and aspirate for definitive diagnosis
- Blast cells in peripheral blood smear (90% of patients)
- Serum chemistries may reveal hyperuricemia.
- Chromosome analysis to determine classification

Treatment

Acute Myelogenous Leukemia

The goal of treatment is to eradicate the leukemic stem cell. Complete remission (CR) is restoration of normal blood counts and fewer than 5% blast cells. The course of therapy is divided into two stages:

1. Induction therapy
   - Cytosine arabinoside continuously for 7 days
   - Anthracycline (e.g., daunorubicin, doxorubicin) for 3 days
   - Bone marrow biopsy on day 14; if leukemic cells are present, begin a second course
   - 20% of AML patients remain in CR; the remainder relapses in 1 to 2 years.
2. Postremission therapy
   - Consolidation: Give high doses of induction therapy drugs for 1 to 2 courses.
   - Intensification: Give different drugs after CR.

Patients who relapse after induction or postremission therapy have a 30% to 60% chance of a second remission. Bone marrow transplant (BMT) for AML is controversial.

Acute Lymphocytic Leukemia

The goal of treatment for ALL is to eradicate leukemic cells from marrow and lymph tissue and residual disease from the central nervous system (CNS). Treatment involves drugs that are more selective to lymphoblasts and less toxic to normal cells. Long-term survival is more favorable with ALL than with AML.

Course of therapy is divided into three stages:

1. Induction therapy
   - Vincristine, prednisone, an anthracycline, cyclophosphamide, and/or asparaginase
   - CR is achieved in 93% of children; only 65% to 85% of adults achieve CR.
2. CNS prophylaxis
   - Intracranial radiation and intrathecal methotrexate

3. Postremission therapy
   - Same drugs as with induction; methotrexate and 6-mercaptopurine may be added.
   - Maintenance therapy often continues for 2 to 3 years.

The outlook is poor for patients who relapse during therapy. There is a better prognosis with BMT if it is performed during the first remission.

CHRONIC MYELOGENOUS LEUKEMIA

Assessment

Patient History and Physical Examination
Approximately 20% of CML patients have no symptoms at diagnosis. Those who are symptomatic often present with the following:

- Left upper quadrant pain, abdominal fullness, and early satiety related to massive splenomegaly
- Malaise, fatigue
- Fever
- Weight loss
- Bone and joint pain

Diagnostic Studies
A complete blood count in the chronic phase usually reveals severe leukocytosis (WBC greater than 100,000/mm^3), anemia, and thrombocytosis. Other laboratory studies reveal high serum B12 levels and low alkaline phosphatase. Bone marrow biopsy demonstrates hyperplasia. Approximately 90% of CML patients have a diagnostic marker, the Philadelphia (Ph^1) chromosome.

Treatment
The only chance for cure of CML is with ablation of the Ph^1 chromosome by high-dose chemotherapy and allogenic BMT. The natural course of CML

has two phases: the chronic phase and, within 30 to 40 months, a terminal phase of accelerated and blastic phases.

Chronic Phase
The standard therapy is oral busulfan or hydroxyurea. Interferon-alfa is also used for untreated or pretreated patients. A new oral drug, STI-571 (Gleevec), has been approved for use in patients with CML myeloid blast crisis, accelerated phase, or chronic phase after failure of interferon treatment. Treatment does not prevent progression to the terminal phase. However, the best chance for cure is allogeneic BMT during the chronic phase.

Terminal Phase
Blastic transformation can be detected 3 to 4 months before clinical signs are evident. Blast crisis requires intensive chemotherapy, similar to agents used for AML. Median survival after onset of the terminal phase is less than 1 year.

CHRONIC LYMPHOCYTIC LEUKEMIA

Assessment

Patient History and Physical Examination
One fourth of individuals with CLL are diagnosed during a routine physical examination. Because CLL is a disease of immunoglobulin-secreting cells, a history of recurrent infections (skin and respiratory) may be elicited. Splenomegaly may be the only clinical finding. Lymphadenopathy occurs in 60% of patients.

Diagnostic Studies
A peripheral blood examination will reveal lymphocytosis with a WBC count greater than 20,000/mm^3 in early disease and a WBC count greater than 100,000/mm^3 in advanced disease. Hypogammaglobulinemia occurs in approximately 50% of patients. Bone marrow biopsy is needed for definitive diagnosis.

PART VI

Treatment

Treatment of CLL consists only of observation until the patient is symptomatic with cytopenias or organomegaly. Symptomatic patients are treated with oral chlorambucil or cyclophosphamide and corticosteroids to control leukocytosis. When the patient no longer responds to steroid therapy, splenectomy and radiation therapy may provide relief of symptoms.

Combination therapy (cyclophosphamide, vincristine, doxorubicin, prednisone) is given for advanced disease. Fludarabine is used in B-cell CLL.

Clinically, hairy cell leukemia is difficult to distinguish from CLL or lymphoma. It is distinguished by massive splenomegaly and pancytopenia, and hairy cells stain positively. Patients are monitored closely. Splenectomy is the treatment of choice for patients with pancytopenia, and interferon-alfa is the treatment of choice when the disease progresses.

Supportive Care

Supportive therapies may improve quality of survival. Nurses play a key role in patient and family education, physical care, psychosocial support, and symptom management. Certain side effects can be ameliorated if detected early and treated promptly.

Neutropenia

An absolute neutrophil count less than 1000/mm^3 is common, and 60% of leukemia patients develop infection.

Common sites of infection

- Pharynx, esophagus
- Lungs
- Anorectal area
- Skin
- Sinuses

The usual signs and symptoms of infection may be absent because of the lack of an inflammatory response. Patients with a fever of more than 100°F require cultures of blood, urine, sputum, and intravenous sites. Additional therapy may include the following:

- Empiric antibiotic therapy until the organism is identified
- Amphotericin B for life-threatening fungal infections and if fever continues 5 to 7 days after the start of antibiotic therapy
- Prophylactic fluconazole to prevent disseminated infections

Prevention of infection focuses on the following actions:

- Maintain the patient's skin integrity, sleep, and nutrition.
- Decrease invasive procedures.
- Provide a private room, and restrict visitors.
- Avoid uncooked foods.
- Encourage meticulous hand washing by the patient and family.
- Do not allow plants or fresh flowers.
- Administer colony-stimulating factors to shorten the period of neutropenia.

Erythrocytopenia
Transfusions of red blood cells are given if there is sudden blood loss or symptomatic anemia.

Thrombocytopenia
There is potential bleeding if the platelet count is less than 50,000/mm^3 and spontaneous bleeding if the platelet count is less than 20,000/mm^3. The first signs of bleeding may be petechiae or ecchymoses on mucous membranes or skin of dependent limbs and oozing from gums, nose, or intravenous site. Random donor platelets may be given to keep the platelet count greater than 20,000/mm^3.

Measures to prevent bleeding
- Maintenance of patient's skin integrity
- Prevention of trauma
- The patient should avoid medications with anticoagulant effects.
- The patient should take stool softeners to prevent straining.

Leukostasis
Patients at risk have a WBC count greater than 50,000/mm³. This occurs most often in patients with ALL. Intracerebral hemorrhage is the most common manifestation. Treatment consists of high doses of cytotoxic drugs to reduce the burden of cells. Leukapheresis and cranial radiation may be used.

Disseminated Intravascular Coagulation
Disseminated intravascualr coagulation (DIC) may occur with any acute leukemia. The correction of DIC depends on successful treatment of leukemia.

Oral Complications
These complications may be a result of disease or therapy. Gingival hypertrophy is associated with massive infiltration by leukemic cells. Stomatitis renders the patient at high risk for oral infection. Routine oral care is of utmost importance.

Cerebellar Toxicity
This CNS toxicity is associated with high-dose cytosine arabinoside (HDCA) (doses > 3 g/m²). There is an increased risk in patients over age 50. Ataxia and nystagmus are early signs. Difficulty with speech and rapid movements are late signs. Toxicity is irreversible if not detected early.

Chapter 49

Liver Cancer

Incidence

Primary and metastatic liver cancers present a significant challenge. Approximately 95% of primary cancer is hepatocellular carcinoma, and its incidence varies greatly throughout the world. Primary liver cancer is the leading cause of death in Africa and Asia, but in the United States it is uncommon. Liver cancer is more prevalent among men than women. The average age of onset is 40 to 60 years.

In the United States, metastatic liver cancer is more common than primary liver cancer because many tumors metastasize to the liver.

Etiology

Primary Liver Cancer

Primary liver cancer has few known etiological factors. The risk factors identified to date are

- hepatitis B or C virus infection,
- environmental carcinogens,
- exposure to aflatoxin,
- cirrhosis,
- schistosomiasis or parasite infections,
- smoking, and
- use of estrogens and androgens.

Metastatic Liver Cancer

Many cancers will eventually metastasize to the liver. The main tumors that migrate to the liver originate from the following primary tumors:

- Breast
- Lung

- Gastrointestinal
- Sarcoma
- Melanoma

Prevention

Measures to prevent liver cancer are few, but vaccination is being explored. Vaccination against hepatitis B is focused on preventing prenatal transmission of the virus. Currently, there is no vaccine for hepatitis C. Chemoprevention may be a future approach, using biological agents such as interferon.

Health education to improve early detection should focus on high-risk populations, such as those who work in food and grain storage occupations and those who share injection needles.

Pathophysiology

Tumors of the liver may be primary tumors or may be secondary tumors that have metastasized from other distant sites. Differentiating whether the tumor is primary or secondary is a critical decision for the selection of the appropriate treatment.

Primary Liver Cancer

The pathology of liver cancer is predominantly hepatocellular (about 90%), and 7% are cholangiocarcinomas. The tumor may be multicentric in origin or start with a single focus. The tumor also is usually soft and highly vascular. The cells will have a macroscopic appearance of nodular, massive, or diffuse.

Metastatic Liver Cancer

Metastatic tumors in the liver are more likely to occur than are primary liver tumors. The liver is the repository for metastatic deposits from nearly all sites. Metastases may occur in the liver as a single mass or as multiple masses.

Progression of Disease

Liver cancer usually progresses and enlarges by direct extension within and around the liver. Tumors typically alter the natural blood flow within the liver. Occlusion of the hepatic circulatory system by tumor leads to necrosis, rupture, and hemorrhage. Ascites and esophageal varices are common sequelae of extensive liver tumor involvement.

Clinical Manifestations

Liver cancer is usually asymptomatic in the early stages.

Common signs of liver cancer that appear with late-stage tumors:

- Upper abdominal pain that is dull and aching
- Continuous pain that begins as dullness and progresses to severe
- Weight loss that exceeds 10%
- Weakness and fatigue
- Intermittent nausea and vomiting
- Fullness in epigastrium
- Constipation or diarrhea
- Anorexia or weight loss
- Jaundice
- Ascites
- Hematemesis
- Hepatic encephalopathy

Assessment

The complete diagnostic assessment of a person with liver cancer includes both subjective and objective information. The patient and family history may reveal risk factors, genetic syndromes, or the contributory diseases listed previously. Physical examination may reveal ascites, jaundice, and a painful, enlarged liver.

PART VI

Diagnostic Studies
More definitive diagnostic studies help define the tumor mass and extent of the disease.

Typical diagnostic studies for liver cancer:

- Abdominal x-ray
- Ultrasound of abdomen
- CT of abdomen, pelvis, and chest
- MRI, PET scan
- Radionuclide scanning
- Selective hepatic arteriography
- Hematological profiles
- Liver function tests
- Tumor marker alpha-fetoprotein (AFP)
- Needle biopsy (only if tumor is considered unresectable)

Treatment
Once a diagnosis is made, the choice of treatment depends on a variety of factors. It is important to know the following:

- Primary or secondary tumor
- Type and extent of tumor
- Concomitant diseases
- Liver function
- Overall patient status

For both primary and metastatic liver cancers, treatment options include surgical resection, liver transplantation, ablative or interstitial therapy, chemotherapy, or radiation therapy. Prior to the initiation of any definitive therapy, the overall health of the patient should be improved if at all possible, including such issues as the following:

- Correcting anemia, clotting deficits, and fluid and electrolyte abnormalities
- Using vitamins A, C, D, and B complex to reduce effect of jaundice
- Relief of pruritus by use of oil-based lotions,

antihistamines, and cholestyramine and by avoiding products that dry the skin

- Improving nutritional status is critical.

Surgery

Primary Liver Cancer

Approximately 15% to 30% of individuals with primary liver cancer are candidates for surgery. Surgery is the most definitive treatment and offers the best chance for cure. Selection of surgical technique depends on tumor size, location, and patient condition.

Resections for liver cancer are as extensive as needed to eradicate the tumor. Major surgical resection procedures include partial or total hepatic lobectomy, also called trisegmentectomy.

The postoperative care following liver resection is principally concerned with the following potential complications:

- Hemorrhage
- Infection
- Subphrenic abscess
- Atelectasis
- Clotting defects
- Biliary fistula
- Transient metabolic changes
- Pneumonia
- Portal hypertension

Cryosurgery

Cryosurgery can be used to treat primary or metastatic liver cancer. It is usually selected as an alternative surgical therapy for unresectable liver tumors. With cryosurgery, tissues are destroyed by using liquid nitrogen applications at subzero temperatures. Following cryosurgery, alkalinization of urine is important to prevent acute tubular necrosis. Pyrexia is typical for about 5 days following therapy.

PART VI

Chemotherapy

Primary Liver Cancer

Systemic chemotherapy for primary liver cancer is administered by two different administration approaches: systemic and regional. Chemotherapy may be the treatment of choice if surgery is not an option.

Doxorubicin remains the standard drug used for systemic treatment, with response rates greater than 20%. Combination immunochemotherapy regimens using multiple agents (cisplatin, interferon, doxorubicin, and 5-fluorouracil [5-FU]) produce response rates of slightly less than 25%. Side effects can be greater than with single-agent therapy.

Liver Metastases

The treatment regimen selected is based on using chemotherapy agents that are proven effective in the management of the specific primary cancer that has metastasized to the liver. 5-FU is the most widely used agent to treat metastatic liver cancer. Typical regimens involve 5-FU, levamisole, and leukovorin. Irinotecan (CPT-11) is considered the next treatment option as second-line therapy.

Regional Therapy

Another alternative method for administering chemotherapy is regional therapy via hepatic artery infusion. Regional therapy is an option for treating unresectable hepatic colorectal metastasis that is isolated to the liver.

Regional therapy provides a high concentration of drug directly to the liver tumor with minimal systemic exposure to the rest of the body. Regional therapy is considered superior to systemic chemotherapy. The major dose limitations are toxicity-related.

Drugs administered via the regional approach are

- 5-FU,

- floxuridine, and
- doxorubicin.

Radiation Therapy

Liver tissue is extremely radiosensitive. Doses are often low because of the extreme sensitivity, and range from 1900 to 3100 cGy. The role of radiation is typically palliation. Radiation is used to treat unresectable liver cancer usually in combination with chemotherapy. Major side effects of radiation to the liver are nausea, vomiting, anorexia, and fatigue.

Alternative Therapies

Chemoembolization

This is a local regional approach to treatment of localized liver tumors. Chemotherapy is mixed with lipid oil to form an emulsion that can cause an impedance to blood flow in the specific area where it is placed. Chemoembolization results in increased exposure of the tumor to the chemotherapy and decreased nutrition to the tumor because the blood supply is embolized. Tumor response rates can be as high as 88%.

Percutaneous Ethanol Injection

This approach is used for small hepatic tumors that are considered unresectable. The injection of ethanol directly into the tumor site generates localized tumor necrosis.

Supportive Care

Most individuals die within 6 months of diagnosis of primary or metastatic liver cancer. It is difficult to detect liver cancer in its early stages; thus, advanced disease is most common.

Advanced liver cancer can result in the following:

- Hepatic encephalopathy
- Severe ascites
- Hepatorenal syndrome

PART VI

- Infection
- Pain
- Bleeding
- Jaundice
- Anorexia and vomiting
- Weight loss

Pain is the most difficult symptom to manage. Pain due to liver cancer tends to worsen at night and is severe. The pain is characteristically aggravated by movement. Aggressive pain management is needed.

Chapter 50

Lung Cancer

Incidence
Lung cancer is the most frequent cause of cancer death in men and women. Cigarette smoking causes 80% to 90% of all lung cancer deaths. Overall cure rates remain a discouraging 14%. Because lung cancer incidence and mortality rates are highest about 35 years after peak exposure, the mortality rates in women will not decline until after the year 2010, when incidence rates plateau.

Etiology
Lung cancer occurs after repeated exposures to substances that cause irritation and inflammation.

Cigarette Smoke
Risk from smoking is determined by multiple factors:
- Number of cigarettes smoked per day: Tobacco smoke is both an initiator and a promoter of cancer. The more cigarettes one smokes per day, the greater the risk.
- Duration of smoking
- Age at which smoking began is related more to duration of smoking than to an increased susceptibility at a younger age.
- Inhalation patterns: The more deeply one inhales, the higher the risk.
- Tar content of cigarettes: Tar is the most carcinogenic compound in cigarettes and causes basal cell hyperplasia, then dysplasia, with displacement of the normal, healthy ciliated and mucus-secreting cells.

Passive Smoke

Passive cigarette smoke, sidestream smoke, or involuntary smoke contains nearly all of the carcinogens contained in mainstream smoke, but, because it is not filtered, contains a greater number of carcinogens. Risk of lung cancer is doubled for persons exposed to 25 or more years of passive smoke during childhood and adolescence. Exposure to environmental tobacco smoke accounts for 30% of all lung cancers.

Asbestos

Asbestos exposure is the most common occupational etiology of lung cancer, causing 3% to 4% of all cases. Asbestos and smoking have a synergistic effect on lung cancer promotion.

Radon

During radioactive decay of uranium, radon products emit heavily ionized alpha particles that, when inhaled, deliver intense radiation to the bronchial epithelium. Radon particles act as both initiators and promoters at the cellular nuclei. Synergy with cigarette smoke is well documented.

Occupational Agents

Increased incidence of lung cancer has been documented in individuals working with arsenic, copper, silica, lead, zinc, gold, chloromethyl ether, diesel exhaust, chromium, coal, hydrocarbons, nickel, ionizing radiation, cadmium, and beryllium.

Indoor Air Pollution

Exposure to carcinogenic cooking oil aerosols, radon, cigarette smoke, building materials, household aerosol products, combustion devices, and other air contaminants increases the risk of lung cancer.

Prevention

Primary Prevention

- If smoking were totally eliminated, 85% of lung cancers would disappear.
- Advertising and marketing strategies target women and children. Consequently, today's death rate from lung cancer in women is 500% higher than that of 1935.
- Over 22 million women in the United States smoke, including 25% of those who are pregnant. Ninety percent of smokers begin smoking before age 20, and most are girls.
- Higher smoking rates are seen in individuals of a lower socioeconomic status, particularly women and male blue-collar workers. Smoking is more common among Blacks.
- Education appears to be inversely related to smoking rates.
- Efforts to prevent smoking must focus on the following:
  - Antismoking education
  - Legislation
  - Taxation of cigarettes

Secondary Prevention

Smoking cessation can reduce the risk for lung cancer in a smoker, depending on how much and how long the person smoked. Smoking cessation strategies are cost effective when more aggressive interventions, such as intensive counseling and the nicotine patch, are used. Health professionals need to emphasize the need for a smoker to quit at every opportunity.

PART VI

Pathophysiology

Cellular Characteristics

Bronchogenic cancers have been grouped into

two major histological categories: small cell lung cancer and the non-small cell lung cancers.

Small Cell Lung Cancer

- Invades the submucosa and is thought to arise from Kulchitsky cells, which are neuroendocrine cells that secrete peptide hormones
- Most are centrally located, developing around a main bronchus.
- Responsible for 25% of all lung cancers
- Small cell lung cancer (SCLC) is an aggressive tumor and is often metastatic at diagnosis.
- Often associated with smoking

Non-Small Cell Lung Cancer
Includes squamous cell carcinoma, adenocarcinoma, and large cell carcinoma

Squamous Cell Carcinoma

- More common in males than females
- Associated with cigarette smoking
- Accounts for 30% of all lung cancers
- Slow growing and longer survival
- Associated with ectopic production of a parathyroid hormone–type substance, causing hypercalcemia

Adenocarcinomas

- Most common of lung cancers in males, females, and nonsmokers.
- Metastasis is common, especially to the brain, liver, bone, and adrenal glands.
- Accounts for 40% of all lung tumors
- Most often present as a single peripheral nodule

Large Cell Carcinoma

- Accounts for 10% to 15% of lung cancers
- Arises as a peripheral nodule and metastasizes early, often to the gastrointestinal tract.

Clinical Manifestations

Clinical manifestations of lung cancer depend on the location of the tumor and the extent of spread. Six percent of patients are asymptomatic at the time of diagnosis. Symptoms may be divided into three categories.

Local–Regional Symptoms
- Cough, dyspnea, wheezing
- Hemoptysis
- Chest pain, stridor, hoarseness
- Hiccups
- Atelectasis and pneumonia
- Pancoast syndrome
- Horner's syndrome
- Pleural and/or pericardial effusion
- Superior vena cava syndrome

Symptoms Due to Extrathoracic Involvement
- Bone bain
- Headache
- Central nervous system disturbances
- Gastrointestinal disturbances
- Jaundice and hepatomegaly
- Abdominal pain

Systemic Symptoms with or without Paraneoplastic Syndromes
- Weakness and fatigue
- Anorexia, cachexia, weight loss
- Anemia
- Symptoms associated with paraneoplastic syndromes

Assessment

After a complete history, a thorough examination of the pulmonary and lymphatic systems is necessary.

PART VI

- Inspection provides information about the pattern of respirations and the symmetry and integrity of the thorax and thoracic configuration.
- Dyspena is a general indication of inadequate respiration.
- Pleuritic chest pain may be manifested by rapid, shallow breathing.
- Intercostal retractions on inspiration indicate obstruction to air inflow.
- Bulging interspaces on expiration are associated with outflow obstruction.
- Stridor indicates extrathoracic airway obstruction.
- Use of accessory muscles for breathing; labored, prolonged expiration; and wheezing may indicate obstruction of intrathoracic airways.
- Clubbing of the fingers; skin changes; weight loss; visible signs of Horner, Pancoast, and SVC syndromes; and joint swelling are noted.
- Palpation may indicate asymmetrical thoracic excursion or tracheal deviation.
- Percussion may determine air and fluid distribution.
- Auscultation determines flow of air and the presence of wheezing, rhonchi, or a friction rub.

Diagnostic Measures
Imaging studies
- Chest radiograph
- Computed tomography
- Positron emission tomography
- Magnetic resonance imaging

Tissue diagnostic studies
- Sputum cytology
- Bronchoscopy
- Fine-needle aspiration
- Mediastinoscopy

- Video-assisted thoracoscopic surgery
- Thoracotomy

Prognostic Indicators

Favorable prognostic indicators in SCLC

- Limited-stage disease
- Metastases limited to a single organ
- Absence of liver or brain metastasis
- Ambulatory performance status
- Female gender
- Normal serum lactic dehydrogenase
- Absence of weight loss
- Immunocompetence
- Presence of the tumor marker neuron-specific enolase (NSE)

Favorable prognostic indicators in non-small cell lung cancer (NSCLC)

- Early-stage cancers respond better to treatment, and patients have longer survival.
- Absence of mediastinal lymph node metastasis
- Stable weight
- Ambulatory performance status
- Female gender
- Normal serum LDH
- Absence of bone or liver metastases

Classification and Staging

Non-Small Cell Lung Cancer
The American Joint Committee on Cancer TMN staging system is recommended for NSCLC.

Small Cell Lung Cancer
Most clinicians use the simple two-stage system designating "limited" or "extensive," because most SCLC patients have metastatic disease at the time of diagnosis.

Treatment

Surgery
Surgery is considered standard curative treatment for stage I and stage II NSCLC. Carefully selected patients with stage IIIa and N2 disease have achieved cure after complete surgical resection. Many surgeons consider individuals with stage IIIB and stage IV lung cancer to be inoperable. Lobectomy or pneumonectomy are surgical procedures for localized disease.

Radiation Therapy
NSCLC responds to radiation and is an option for patients who are not surgical candidates. Postoperative radiation therapy is the standard of care for selected stage IIIa patients and for patients with unresectable stage III disease.

For patients with SCLC, radiation and chemotherapy are standard therapies for limited-stage disease. Prophylactic cranial irradiation (PCI) in limited-stage SCLC is under investigation. Researchers contend that while PCI may reduce brain recurrence, it does not improve overall survival, and the associated morbidity does not justify brain irradiation unless a metastatic brain lesion develops.

Radiation is commonly used to palliate symptoms of metastatic disease, especially for patients with bone metastases or spinal cord compression and for individuals with superior vena cava syndrome.

Chemotherapy
Non-small cell lung cancer

- 50% to 75% of all patients with NSCLC will present with nonresectable or metastatic disease. Eighty percent of those patients with resectable disease will relapse and be candidates for chemotherapy.
- A survival advantage has been demonstrated in stage III individuals treated with a cisplatin-based chemotherapy regimen followed by radiation.

- Other chemotherapy regimens include irinote-can, paclitaxel, docetaxel, vinorelbine, and gemcitabine.

Small cell lung cancer

- Chemotherapy with or without radiation therapy is the mainstay of treatment for many years.
- Typical combinations of treatment include cyclophosphamide, doxorubicin, vincristine (CAV); etoposide, cisplatin; oral etoposide and cisplatin; and carboplatin and etoposide.
- Other chemotherapy agents active in SCLC include gemcitabine, paclitaxel, docetaxel, topotecan, and irinotecan.

Supportive Care

Supportive care is of utmost importance due to the distressing physical symptoms.

- Cough may result from stimulation of irritant receptors in the bronchial mucosa through tumor infiltration, or hypersecretion of mucus.
- Hemoptysis is caused by erosion of the pulmonary vasculature by tumor.
- Dyspnea and the sensation of smothering is common in advanced lung cancer. It may be associated with pleural effusion.
- Pain is experienced by most individuals with lung cancer and may be caused by mediastinal extension of tumor, pleural effusions, bronchial obstruction, or infection.
- Fatigue and weakness have been the most commonly reported symptoms in lung cancer.
- Gastrointestinal disturbances, including nausea and vomiting, anorexia, and cachexia are common in patients with lung cancer.
- Psychosocial issues, including fear and anxiety, are common among individuals with lung cancer and have been associated with high degrees of suffering.

PART VI

Chapter 51

Multiple Myeloma

Incidence
Multiple myeloma represents 1% of hematological malignancies. The onset of multiple myeloma is late, with peak incidence between ages 50 and 70. Multiple myeloma is more common among African Americans than all other racial groups. There is predominance in incidence among males.

Etiology
The exact etiology of multiple myeloma is unknown, although a variety of risk factors have been noted.

Risk Factors
- Genetic linkage among close relatives
- Chronic low-level exposure to radiation
- Chronic antigenic stimulation due to recurrent infections, drug allergies
- Occupational exposure to wood, textiles, rubber, metal, petroleum, and herbicides
- Human herpes virus-8 infection

Pathophysiology
Multiple myeloma is characterized by an overproduction of one specific immunoglobulin, designated IgM, or M protein (i.e., myeloma or malignant protein). About 80% to 90% of multiple myeloma patients have evidence of the aberrant M protein in their serum. Although an excessive amount of IgM immunoglobulin is produced, the body is unable to produce enough antibodies necessary for maintaining humoral immunity.

Cytokines, specifically interleukin-6, have been identified as major growth factors in the development of multiple myeloma. The disease affects the hematological, skeletal, renal, and nervous system.

Clinical Manifestations

Multiple myeloma has a long prodromal, indolent, or asymptomatic period, yet once symptoms appear, an untreated individual can have a median survival of 7 months. Likewise, standard therapy can extend survival for 2 to 3 years.

The most frequent symptom of multiple myeloma at presentation is bone pain. Symptoms of active disease include the following:

Skeletal Involvement

- 68% to 80% of patients present with destructive, painful osteolytic lesions.
- Hypercalcemia occurs in 20% to 40% of patients.
- Pathological fractures are common.
- Mobility decreases and ability in activities of daily living diminishes.
- Bony lesions can be of three types:
  - Solitary osteolytic lesion
  - Diffuse osteoporosis
  - Multiple discrete osteolytic lesions ("punched out" or "cannon ball" lesions)
- Eventually skeletal involvement can lead to
  - compression fractures of spine,
  - refractory hypercalcemia, and
  - death from neurological sequelae or severe hypercalcemia and renal failure.

Infection

- 50% to 70% of patients die of bacterial infections.

- The most common sites of infection are the respiratory and urinary tracts.
- A biphasic pattern of infection is common, with *Streptococcus pneumoniae* and *Haemophilus influenzae* infections occurring early in the disease (within 8 months) and nonencapsulated gram-negative bacilli and *Staphylococcus aureus* infections occurring later.
- Infections result from
  - deficiency in the immunoglobulin response,
  - neutropenia associated with bone marrow suppression, and
  - qualitative defects in neutrophil and complement system function.

Bone Marrow Involvement
- Normocytic, normochromic anemia is found in more than 60% of patients at initial diagnosis.
- An M-protein coating on erythrocytes causes hemolysis and capillary sludging.
- Bleeding can be caused by decreased platelets, M protein's effect on clotting factors, or by coating of platelets with immunoglobulins.

Renal Insufficiency
- 50% of patients will eventually develop renal failure, while 15% of those will die of renal insufficiency.
- Multiple myeloma produces intrinsic renal lesions associated with renal failure called myeloma kidney.
- Bence-Jones proteins that develop in multiple myeloma are toxic to the renal epithelium.
- Large amounts of amyloid deposits can cause another type of renal lesion in about 30% of patients.

Assessment

Physical examination findings may include bone pain, change in mobility, and signs of cord compression.

The most common diagnostic measures

- Bone marrow biopsy to check for greater than 10% plasma cells
- Serum protein electrophoresis to check for presence of M protein
- Serum chemistry to determine hypercalcemia or renal insufficiency
- Complete blood count to rule out anemia, thrombocytopenia
- Skeletal survey to check for osteolytic bone lesions

Classification and Staging

The Durie-Salmon system of stages I to III is commonly used. Staging of multiple myeloma integrates the clinical and laboratory findings and estimated total body myeloma mass.

Treatment

Patients with indolent, asymptomatic multiple myeloma are usually not treated. Once symptoms occur (anemia, hypercalcemia, pain), standard therapy is initiated. Common treatment approaches include chemotherapy and radiation.

Chemotherapy

- Melphalan and prednisone are standard first-line therapy for multiple myeloma.
  - The response rate to chemotherapy is 50%, and survival time is usually 24 to 36 months.
  - Melphalan is given for 4 days, along with prednisone for 7 days, and the cycle is repeated every 4 weeks.
  - The patient is monitored closely for signs of renal impairment.

PART VI

- The side effects of this regimen are quite tolerable.
- If multiple myeloma is unresponsive to the initial chemotherapy, the dose of melphalan may be escalated until a response is achieved.

- Another common first-line chemotherapy protocol for multiple myeloma is the combination of vincristine, doxorubicin, and dexamethasone (VAD), which may be used as the first-line therapy and for resistant or refractory disease.
- Side effects can be more significant than those with standard therapy, which is why this more aggressive therapy is not selected first. Response rates may be higher than with standard therapy (65%–75%).
- During therapy, clinicians must closely monitor and anticipate the following:
  - Total cumulative dose of doxorubicin
  - Signs of steroid toxicity
    - Severe dyspepsia
    - Fluid and sodium retention
    - Myopathy
    - Pancreatitis
    - Hyperglycemia
    - Steroid psychosis
  - Signs of neurological toxicity
  - Bone marrow suppression
  - Hepatic toxicity

If drug resistance emerges and tumor response is negligible, then cyclophosphamide therapy can be used. Overall, 30% to 40% of patients will not respond to first-line therapy; thus, second-line therapies are commonly used, with response rates of 70%.

Interferon
Interferon stimulates the host cells to inhibit plasma cell and inhibit myeloma stem-cell growth. Interferon has been used as neoadjuvant

therapy for untreated patients and as an adjunct after standard first-line chemotherapy to prolong tumor response and extend survival time.

Radiation
Multiple myeloma is highly radioresponsive. Hemibody irradiation has been used in select situations for treatment of refractory or advanced myeloma. Radiation is also used to palliate bone lesions and control pain.

Bone Marrow Transplantation
Both bone marrow transplantation and peripheral stem cell support have been used in the treatment of multiple myeloma.

Long-Term Sequelae
Aggressive treatment of multiple myeloma can result in latent or long-term effects. Among those effects is treatment-related acute leukemia. The leukemia usually develops many years (10 to 20) after primary therapy. Most patients who develop leukemia have a dismal prognosis of 4 to 8 months.

Supportive Care
The chronic nature of this disease requires ongoing symptom management.

- Pain from multiple myeloma is usually caused by bony involvement. Aggressive pain management approaches, positioning, braces, supports, and massages can help.
- Mental status changes can result from hypercalcemia, hyperviscosity, or drug toxicity. It is important to closely assess the patient to prevent injury.
- Infection is a common cause of death. Early recognition and measures to prevent infection are needed.
- Measures to prevent pooling of secretions in the lungs and to increase gas exchange can

PART VI

minimize the effects of multiple myeloma on the lungs.

- Decreased physical activity and medications can result in constipation. Frequently assess the patient's activity level and dietary intake to detect any changes.

- Renal insufficiency can be prevented or minimized by providing adequate hydration, administration of allopurinol, and close monitoring for signs of urinary tract infection.

Chapter 52

Non-Hodgkin's Lymphoma

Incidence

The incidence of non-Hodgkin's lymphoma (NHL) is escalating in the United States. It is now the fifth most common cancer in males and females. NHL is diagnosed nearly six times as often as Hodgkin's disease, and the death rate is 13 times greater. The incidence is higher in males than in females and in the white population more than blacks. The average age of occurrence is the fifth decade.

Etiology

A variety of etiological factors have been implicated:

- Viral infections
- Genetic abnormalities
- Exposure to pesticides, fertilizers, and chemicals

Pathophysiology

At present, the sequence of events that explains the transformation of a normal lymphocyte into a lymphomatous cell is unknown. Cytogenic analysis of both B-cell and T-cell origin in NHL reveal chromosomal abnormalities.

Clinical Manifestations

NHL can involve almost any organ or tissue. Approximately 80% of patients present with advanced disease (stage III or IV), reflected by the following:

- Painless, generalized lymphadenopathy and "B" symptoms

- Fever
- Nightsweats
- Weight loss
- Gastrointestinal symptoms
  - Pain
  - Abdominal mass
  - Anorexia
- Lung infiltration
  - Cough
  - Dyspnea
  - Chest pain
  - Pleural effusion
- Superior vena cava syndrome
- Bone, liver, and brain manifestations

Assessment

A careful history and physical examination should be precise in evaluating clinical manifestations and length of time present. Diagnostic measures include

- biopsy to confirm histopathology,
- cytogenetics analysis, and
- immunohistochemistry stains.

Classification and Staging

The classification of NHL is complex, and numerous systems (Working Formulation, Rappaport System, Real Classification) are used. In spite of the various classifications, the concept of low-, intermediate-, and high-grade lymphomas is useful for clinical purposes.

Low-Grade Lymphomas

- Occur in older individuals (median age, 55)
- Affect males and females equally
- A majority of patients are asymptomatic.
- The usual presenting problem is painless lymphadenopathy.

- Slow growing, with median survival of 7 to 9 years

Intermediate-Grade Lymphomas
- Uncommon tumors with a follicular architecture and predominantly large lymphocytes
- Have an aggressive clinical course
- Most patients have advanced disease at the time of diagnosis.

High-Grade Lymphomas
- These aggressive lymphomas exhibit rapid growth.
- Without treatment, survival is less than 18 months.
- With treatment, there is potential for cure because they respond to chemotherapy.
- Prognosis is influenced by five pretreatment characteristics
  - Age (over 60 versus under 60)
  - Extent of disease (stage I or II versus stage III or IV)
  - Performance status (0–1 versus 2 or more)
  - Number of extranodal sites (none versus one or more)
  - LDH level (normal versus elevated)

Staging work-up determines extent of disease, tumor mass, and potential complications. NHL occurs in many locations and requires numerous studies for staging. Patients are classified according to the Ann Arbor–Cotswolds staging system.

Treatment
Treatment depends on histology, extent of disease, and performance status.

Low-Grade Lymphomas
Some physicians hold off treatment until symptoms appear. When symptoms develop, treatment includes radiation therapy or chemotherapy. An

PART VI

alternate approach is intensive combination chemotherapy regimens. Rituximab, a monoclonal antibody, is used for the treatment of relapsed or refractory low-grade NHL.

Intermediate and High-Grade Lymphomas

Aggressive combination chemotherapy is the treatment of choice for intermediate- and high-grade lymphomas. CHOP (cyclophosphamide, doxorubicin, vincristine, and prednisone) is a commonly used regimen.

Supportive Care

Nursing care is related to radiation and chemotherapeutic side effects, which is covered in Chapters 10 and 11. Nurses play a pivotal role in providing emotional support and symptom management, and in rehabilitating the cured patient to return to a healthy lifestyle.

Chapter 53

Ovarian Cancer

Incidence
Approximately 23,400 new cases and 13,000 deaths of ovarian cancer occur annually. Ovarian cancer is the most common cause of death from gynecological cancers and the fourth leading cause of cancer death in women. It is estimated that 1 in 70 women will develop ovarian cancer. The disease occurs most often between ages 40 and 70.

Etiology
Hormonal, environmental, and genetic factors play a role in the development of ovarian cancer (Table 53.1).

Pathophysiology
Cellular Characteristics
Epithelial tumors constitute 85% to 90% of ovarian cancers. Mutations of the *p53* gene have been identified in 30% to 79% of epithelial tumors.

Table 53.1 Factors in the Development of Ovarian Cancer

Risk Factors	Preventive Factors
Nulliparity	Parity
Use of infertility drugs	Lactation
Pelvic inflammatory disease	Oral contraceptives
Low serum gonadotropin	Tubal ligation
Living in industralized Western countries	Oophorectomy
Family history of breast or ovarian cancer	
Being of Jewish descent	

Germ-cell or sex-cord stromal cell tumors constitute the remainder.

Progression of Disease
Ovarian cancer commonly spreads by direct extension. It penetrates the capsule of the ovary and invades the structures next to it (i.e., uterus, fallopian tubes, bladder, rectosigmoid colon, and pelvic peritoneum). Peritoneal seeding occurs because of continuous circulation of the peritoneal fluid in the peritoneal cavity. Disease spreads to the liver, diaphragm, bladder, or intestines by this route.

Prognostic Factors
Prognostic indicators are age, performance status, and abnormality of oncogenes such as *p53*, *MYC*, *RAS*, and *ERB-2*.

Clinical Manifestations
Approximately 75% of ovarian cancer patients have metastatic disease at diagnosis. Death is often secondary to intraabdominal tumor dissemination that produces bowel and mesentery malfunction and alteration. Common signs and symptoms of ovarian cancer are listed in Table 53.2.

Assessment
During physical examination, the presence of an ovarian mass is the most significant finding. An

Table 53.2 Signs and Symptoms of Ovarian Cancer

Early Signs	Late Signs
Lower abdominal pressure: discomfort, pain	Ascites
Abdominal distention	Pleural effusion
Change in bowel or bladder habits	Anorexia
Early satiety	Nausea or vomiting
Indigestion, dyspepsia	Abdominal, pelvic, ovarian, omental mass
Back pain	

immobile, painless, irregular mass is suspicious of ovarian cancer. In premenopausal women, enlarged ovaries are common due to cysts. If a mass enlarges during the period of observation, further evaluation is needed.

Diagnostic studies typically include

- pelvic examination,
- CA-125 assay,
- transvaginal ultrasound,
- CT scan,
- barium enema or colposcopy, and
- chest x-ray.

Classification and Staging

The International Federation of Obstetrics and Gynecology (FIGO) staging system is universally used. Stage I disease has a 5-year survival of 85%. Stage IV has a survival of 18%.

Treatment

Surgical Staging

- Evaluation of all peritoneal surfaces
- Evaluation of subdiaphragmatic surfaces
- Multiple biopsies
- Palpation of all abdominal organs and surfaces

Cytoreduction of Tumor Mass

Surgical procedures used to remove visible tumor to the extent possible

- Total abdominal hysterectomy
- Bilateral salpingoophorectomy
- Peritoneal cytology
- Omentectomy

Secondary cytoreductive surgery used at time of relapse is controversial. Palliative surgery is used when bowel obstruction occurs.

Common problems following surgery for ovarian cancer

- Bleeding/hemorrhage

PART VI

- Thromboembolic event
- Infection/sepsis
- Fluid and electrolyte imbalance
- Atelectasis/pneumonia
- Bowel and bladder dysfunction

The treatment approach depends on the stage of disease.

Early-Stage Disease

Early-stage disease is divided according to favorable risk or unfavorable risk.

Favorable or low-risk disease requires no further treatment beyond initial surgery.

Unfavorable-risk disease has a high rate of relapse and should receive adjuvant chemotherapy. Cisplatin, cyclophosphamide, and/or carboplatin are most often used in combination therapy.

Advanced Disease

Advanced disease is routinely managed with a combination of chemotherapy and radiation. Cytoreductive surgery is possible in only 50% of cases. Chemotherapy regimens use anthracyclines, platinum-based compounds, and the taxanes.

Maintenance Therapy

With primary therapy and complete remission achieved, maintenance or consolidation therapy can be used to decrease relapse rate, although this approach is controversial.

Maintenance therapy involves

- high-dose chemotherapy,
- intraperitoneal therapy,
- radiotherapy (whole abdominal radiation), and
- prolonged chemotherapy.

Supportive Care

Major problems in caring for women with advanced recurrent disease:

Ascites
- One-third present with ascites, and two-thirds have ascites at death.
- Paracentesis may provide temporary relief.
- Intraperitoneal chemotherapy is used for obliteration of ascites.

Intestinal Obstruction
- The patient will have colicky abdominal pain and abdominal distention.
- Decompression of the bowel with a nasogastric tube or bowel rest may be used initially.
- Analgesics, antiemetics, and anticholinergics are prescribed to manage pain, nausea, and vomiting.
- Surgery is the last option.

Malnutrition
- Anorexia and cachexia both lead to malnutrition.
- Corticosteroids, appetite stimulants, metachlopromide, and megestrol acetate may be used to stimulate the appetite.
- Aggressive nutrition (oral, enteral, TPN) may be necessary.

Lymphedema
- Lower extremity involvement occurs from blockage of pelvic nodes, which requires primary treatment of the tumor.
- Decongestive physiotherapy (massage, exercises, compressions)

Pleural Effusion
- Effusion will develop in 25% to 30% of patients.
- Dyspnea, pain, fever, and cough are common presenting symptoms.
- Treatment includes thoracentesis, pleurodesis, oxygen, and morphine.

Chapter 54

Pancreatic Cancer

Incidence

Pancreatic cancer is the fifth leading cause of cancer deaths in the United States and accounts for 2% of all cancers. The 5-year survival rate is only 3%. Fewer than 20% of affected individuals will be alive 1 year after diagnosis. Pancreatic cancer is difficult to detect or diagnose before the cancer has advanced.

Peak incidence occurs between ages 60 and 80 and is equal in incidence among males and females. There is a slightly higher incidence among Blacks, Jewish individuals, and persons living in industrialized nations.

Etiology

Environmental factors are thought to be most relevant etiological factors.

Risk Factors

- Age greater than 60 years
- Genetics
  - Activation of oncogene *K-RAS*
  - Inactivation of suppressor genes (*p16*)
- Tobacco use
- Exposure to radiation
- Diet high in carbohydrate, meat, and salt
- Obesity
- Occupational exposure
- Chemists, coal/gas, metal workers, dye industry
- Diabetes
- Chronic pancreatitis

There is a protective effect from a diet high in fresh fruits and vegetables.

Pathophysiology

Pancreatic cancer is predominantly an adenocarcinoma arising from the cells lining the pancreatic duct. About 90% of tumors arise from the endocrine pancreas. Tumors occur in the head of the pancreas in 60% to 70% of cases.

Pancreatic tumors grow slowly, with late signs of pathology. At diagnosis, 90% of cases have perineural invasion, and 70% to 80% have lymphatic spread. Most common sites of metastases are direct extension into adjacent organs: duodenum, retroperitoneum, celiac plexus, kidney, and left adrenal gland.

Clinical Manifestations

Early signs are vague and contribute to a delay in diagnosis. Weight loss and abdominal pain are the most prominent signs. Weight loss is accelerated by pain, anorexia, nausea, vomiting, and malabsorption can lead to diarrhea, constipation, steatorrhea, and weakness. Depending on the site of the tumor, clinical signs may vary.

Head of Pancreas Tumors

These tumors manifest signs earlier than in other parts of the pancreas. The classic triad of symptoms is pain, weight loss, and jaundice.

- Pain
    - In epigastric region
    - Dull and intermittent
    - Ameliorated by sitting in fetal position
- Profound weight loss
- Jaundice
    - Presenting symptom in 80% of cases
    - Jaundice with pain is more common than painless jaundice.
- Patients complain of emotional disturbances and irritability.

PART VI

Body of Pancreas Tumors

These tumors manifest symptoms late in advanced stages and include

- severe, excruciating epigastric pain, causing vomiting;
- splenomegaly; and
- vomiting and weight loss.

Tail of Pancreas Tumors

- Mimic other diseases
- Generalized weakness
- Severe upper abdominal pain
- Indigestion, anorexia, and weight loss

Assessment

Because the pancreas is an inaccessible organ, physical examination usually reveals little diagnostic information. A palpable liver is found in 50% of cases.

Diagnostic studies

- Radiological studies: ultrasound, CT scan, endoscopic retrograde cholangiopancreatography (ERCP), angiography, endoscopic ultrasound, PET, percutaneous fine-needle aspiration
- Laboratory: chemistry profiles, tumor markers (CA 19-9, CA 50, CA 494)

Classification and Staging

There is no consensus on the approach to staging. The TNM system of staging and classification is widely used.

Treatment

Recent reports on surgical outcomes are encouraging, and the outlook on treating pancreatic cancer is improving. If cure is possible, then radical therapy should be used. Palliation is the goal if the disease is advanced. Surgery, chemotherapy, and radiation are all used to treat pancreatic cancer. Multimodal therapy is being studied to determine whether survival is extended.

Surgical Approaches for Cure or Control

- Pancreatoduodenectomy (Whipple procedure)
  - Resection of distal stomach, pancreas to superior mesenteric vein, duodenum, proximal jejunum, distal common duct, and gallbladder
  - Most commonly performed operation for pancreatic cancer and for tumor of head of pancreas
  - A modified approach, pylorus-preserving pancreaticoduodenectomy, is preferred by some.
  - Pancreatic fistula and delayed gastric emptying are complications.
- Extended (radical) pancreatectomy
  - Resection of entire pancreas, duodenum, gastric antrum, bile duct, gallbladder, spleen, and nodes
  - Lymph node involvement is an important prognostic indicator.
  - No published survival advantage over Whipple procedure
- Total pancreatectomy
  - En bloc resection, including antrum, common duct, gallbladder, pancreas, jejunum, duodenum, and nodes
  - Patients develop endocrine and exocrine insufficiency.
  - Eliminates any questionable tumor margins; offers no survival advantage
- Distal pancreatectomy
  - Used for early-stage tumors of body and tail
  - Resection of only involved pancreas and nodes

PART VI

Surgical Approaches for Palliation

Palliative approaches are used in over 90% of cases. Obstructive jaundice, duodenal obstruction, and pain are common symptoms needing aggressive palliation. Surgical palliation procedures include measures to decompress obstructed areas and relieve pain:

- Cholecystojejunostomy
- Choledochojejunostomy
- Pancreatojejunostomy
- Biliary bypass procedures
- Percutaneous or endoscopic gastro-enterostomy
- Biliary stents
- Chemical splanchnicectomy (alcohol nerve block) for pain

Postoperative Care

To minimize serious complications, care focuses on prevention of the following:

- Hemorrhage
- Hypovolemia
- Hypotension
- Pulmonary complications
- Exocrine and endocrine alterations
  - Endocrine function can be regulated with insulin.
  - Exocrine function can result in malabsorption syndromes.
  - Nutritional therapy, pancreatic enzyme supplements, and lipase administration may be needed.
- Diet therapy
  - Low-fat, high-carbohydrate foods; small meals; restriction of caffeine and alcohol

Chemotherapy

Chemotherapy is used as adjuvant therapy with limited results. Combination chemotherapy and radiation has shown marginal improvement in palliation.

Single agents alone are ineffective. Combination therapy involves 5-fluorouracil (5-FU), ifosfamide, mitomycin, doxorubicin, streptozotocin, and gemcitabine.

Radiation Therapy

This therapy is used for both palliative and curative external therapy. A limitation to effectiveness is the large volume of tissue to be irradiated and the limited tolerance of surrounding organs. Combinations of radiotherapy and chemotherapy (5-FU) are being used successfully to increase survival time following surgical resection.

Supportive Care

Most common measures

- Continuous administration of pain relief medications
- Nutritional support via oral feedings, supplemental mixtures, antiemetic therapy, feeding tube, and pancreatic enzyme replacements
- Relief of jaundice using cholestyramine and lotions and avoiding soaps
- Relief of obstruction via percutaneous transhepatic biliary drainage

Chapter 55

....

Prostate Cancer

Incidence

Prostate cancer is the most commonly diagnosed solid tumor in American males and the second leading cause of cancer-related deaths. Black males have the highest incidence of prostate cancer, with a mortality rate twice that of white males.

Etiology

The cause of prostate cancer is unknown, but risk factors include the following:

- Age: The incidence after age 50 increases on a yearly basis to reach approximately 1000 cases per 100,000 males age 65 to 69. By age 80 to 84, the incidence per 100,000 males is greater than 3000.

- Lifestyle factors include nutrition and exposure to carcinogens. High fat consumption and a diet high in animal fat may alter the hormonal environment. Exposure to carcinogens such as cigarette smoke, cadmium, or zinc may play a role.

- Bilateral vasectomy may increase the risk of prostate cancer.

- Heredity-linked prostate cancer is characterized by an early onset of disease.

- Black males have the highest incidence of prostate cancer in the world, which may be related to their reluctance to participate in screening, a variance in androgen levels, or multiple genetic changes.

Pathophysiology

A majority of prostate cancers are adenocarcinomas. All prostate cancers arise from glandular epithelial cells. Premalignant changes in prostate tissue is termed *prostatic intraepithelial neoplasia* (PIN), and may be present for 10 or more years before cancer is diagnosed.

Clinically important cancers include features such as large tumor volume; Gleason grade 3 to 5 (moderate to poor differentiation); an invasive, proliferative pattern of growth; elevated PSA; and origination in the peripheral zone.

Prostate cancer is usually characterized by a slow pattern of growth, locally, along tissue planes. Perineural invasion may accompany capsular invasion. When lymphatic metastases occur, they may involve the obturator, presacral, presciatic, internal, and external iliac nodes. Distant sites of metastasis include the lungs, bladder, and liver.

Clinical Manifestations

Prostate cancer is usually asymptomatic in its early stages. As the disease progresses, patients may present with urinary tract obstructive symptoms, such as frequency, incomplete bladder emptying, hesitancy, nocturia, and urgency.

Advanced prostate cancer may present with ureteral obstruction, hydronephrosis, or back pain due to possible vertebral body metastases, with the potential for spinal cord compression.

Assessment

Screening for prostate cancer involves digital rectal examination (DRE), analysis of prostate-specific antigen (PSA), and, if necessary, transrectal ultrasound.

Once a diagnosis of prostate cancer is made, the patient may undergo the following diagnostic tests:

- PSA will reflect the severity of the patient's disease and will be used periodically to evaluate disease response to therapy and to monitor the patient for cancer relapse.

PART VI

- DRE involves palpation of the prostate gland, with special attention to the anterior and midline of the prostate.
- TRUS is an evaluation of the gland using transrectal ultrasound and is useful to evaluate the extent of localized prostate cancer.
- CT, bone scan, and MRI

Classification and Staging

Prostate cancer is most commonly staged according to the American Urologic Association system or the TNM system.

- Stage A refers to disease that is asymptomatic: Ten-year survival is 95%.
- Stage B1 refers to disease in less than both lobes of the gland: Ten-year survival is 80%.
- Stage B2 involves both lobes of the prostate: Ten-year survival is 80%.
- Stage C disease indicates that cancer has invaded into or beyond the prostate capsule: Ten-year survival is 60%.
- Stage D cancer involves nodes only: Ten-year survival is 40%.
- Stage D where cancer has metastasized: Ten-year survival is 10%.

Treatment

Treatment is controversial and varies depending on the aggressive nature of the disease and whether it is considered to be clinically important.

- Watchful waiting or periodic observation may be appropriate for early-stage disease and as a treatment option for older men.
- Radical prostatectomy may be appropriate for younger men in good health with localized tumors. Complications may include impotence and urinary incontinence.
- External beam radiotherapy or prostatic brachytherapy that involves the placement of

radioactive seeds directly into the prostate may be curative treatment for localized disease. Either may also be used for palliation for advanced disease. Common side effects include proctitis, urinary frequency, cystitis, and diarrhea, as well as incontinence and impotency.

- Endocrine manipulation is usually used as palliation to reduce tumor size.
- Methods
  - Bilateral orchiectomy
  - Hormonal agents such as flutamide, leuprolide, and goserelin acetate
    - Complications of hormonal manipulation include hot flashes, nausea and vomiting, edema, decreased libido, and erectile impotence.
- Chemotherapy plays a limited role for advanced, hormonally unresponsive prostate cancer. Potential agents include oral etoposide or oral estramustine.

Supportive Care
Patients with advanced disease may require nursing intervention and symptom management for the following:

- Bone pain may require combination analgesics and precautions to prevent fractures.
- Management of leg and scrotal edema with scrotal elevation, diuretics, compression stockings, and prevention of lymphedema.
- Catheterization for bladder obstruction
- Monitoring for spinal cord compression, pulmonary embolism, or disseminated intravascular coagulation

PART VI

Chapter 56
∙∙∙∙∙∙∙∙∙∙∙∙∙∙

Skin Cancer

Incidence
Skin cancer accounts for approximately one-third of all diagnosed cancers. There are more than one million cases of basal cell carcinomas and squamous cell carcinomas detected annually. The increased incidence is related to cumulative sun-exposure behaviors.

The annual incidence of the more serious form of skin cancer malignant melanoma (MM) is rising annually, from a risk of 1 out of 1500 to 1 out of 75 persons annually. It is increasing worldwide at a faster rate than any other cancer. The mortality rate continues to increase. Nonmelanoma skin cancers (NMSCs) occur more often but have a lower mortality rate than malignant melanomas.

There are two groups of NMSCs:

1. Basal cell carcinoma (BCC)
   - Most common skin cancer in whites
   - More frequent in men
   - Least aggressive type
2. Squamous cell carcinoma (SCC)
   - More frequent in men
   - More aggressive than BCC

The other, more severe group of skin cancers is malignant melanomas.

- Most are cutaneous melanomas (CM)
- Primarily occur in whites
- More frequent in men

Etiology
The etiology of skin cancer is multifactorial. Different skin cancers are associated with different risk factors (Table 56.1).

Table 56.1 Risk Factors for Skin Cancer

Risk Factor	Risk for NMSC	Risk for MM
Actinic keratoses	+	+
Congenital nevus		+
Family history of melanoma		+
History of NMSC in a first-degree relative	+	
History of three or more blistering sunburns before age of 20	+	+
Increasing age	+	+
Ionizing radiation	+	
Large number of dysplastic or melanocytic nevi		+
Male gender	+	+
Personal history of BCC, MM, or SCC	+	+
Red or blond hair	+	+
Skin color, tendency to freckle	+	+

Prevention

Primary and secondary prevention are both important in regard to skin cancer. Primary preventive strategies include

- proper application and use of sunscreens,
- wearing protective clothing, and
- decreasing ultraviolet radiation (UVR) exposure.

Secondary preventive strategies include

- risk assessment,
- practice of monthly self-skin examination, and
- annual professional examination.

Pathophysiology

Nonmelanoma Skin Cancers

BCC results when a malignant transformation of the basal cells occurs. Its nature is slow-growing and nonmetastatic. There is a 95% cure rate with complete excision of the primary BCC.

SCC arises from malignant transformation of keratinocytes. It can rapidly progress and metastasizes, depending on location, depth, and size of the tumor. Overall 5-year survival rate is 90%, and the metastatic rate is 3% to 6%.

Malignant Melanoma

Most MMs occur in cutaneous sites after malignant transformation of melanocytes. MMs exhibit two growth phases: radial and vertical. There is a risk of local recurrence, and distant metastases involve skin, lymph nodes, lungs, liver, brain, bone, and small intestine.

A poor prognosis is associated with deep lesions; lesions on the trunk, head, neck, heels, and palms; and nodal involvement. Females appear to have a better prognosis than do males.

Clinical Manifestations

Nonmelanoma Skin Cancer

- Nonhealing sore or ulcer
- Scaling red or pink patch that does not heal
- Enlarging pink papule or nodule
- New nodule with or without scaling, erosion, ulceration, or crusting
- Pearly papule with telangiectasia

Common sites include the face, back of hands, foreams, ears, lower lip, and trunk of the body.

Malignant Melanoma

- New pigmented or unpigmented nevus
- A nevus that is asymmetrical

- A preexisting lesion that developed irregular borders
- A nevus that is persistently itchy, tender, or bleeding
- A nevus that has grown to 6 mm or greater than 6 mm
- May be found anywhere on the body

Assessment
A risk assessment and thorough history are the first steps. The mainstay for the early detection of both NMSC and MM is the physical examination. Biopsy of the suspicious lesion is necessary for histological examination. Patients diagnosed with MM should undergo diagnostic testing to rule out metastases.

Classification and Staging
The TNM staging system is used for NMSC. Two systems are used to describe MMs: Clark's level and Breslow's measurement.

Treatment
Treatment selection depends on tumor type, location, size, growth pattern, patient age, and general health.

Nonmalignant Melanoma Skin Cancers
Surgical Excision
- Can be performed for any NMSC
- Allows rapid healing
- Provides good cosmetic results

Mohs' Micrographic Surgery
- Used for tumors that are recurrent, those with indistinct margins, and in high risk areas (nose, ear)
- Complex and specialized technique

Electrosurgery
- Useful for removal of distinct, superficial, or nodular BCCs

PART VI

Cryotherapy

- Involves liquid nitrogen to freeze and thaw tissue; leads to tumor necrosis
- Used for superficial SCC

Radiotherapy

- Used for small lesions that are difficult to excise (corner of nose, eyelid, lip, and canthus)

Chemotherapy

- Topical and intralesional 5-FU has been used to treat BCCs.
- Retinoids have caused regression of skin cancers.

Malignant Melanoma

Surgery

- Surgical excision should be wide and include disease-free margins.
- Lymph node dissection remains very controversial.
- Lymphatic mapping identifies those patients who would benefit from selective lymph node dissection.

Chemotherapy

- Metastatic melanoma is resistant to chemotherapeutic agents.
- DTIC as a single agent or a combination regimen of DTIC, BCNU, cisplatin, and tamoxifen has shown some response in treating metastatic MM.

Radiation Therapy

- Treatment of choice for patients who cannot undergo surgery
- May be used as an adjuvant with surgical excision in high-recurring tumors
- Often used for palliation

Immunotherapy

- Nonspecific immunotherapy agents are used to stimulate the immune system.

- Interferon
- Interleukin-2
- Bacille Calmette-Guérin
- Specific immunotherapy agents target the tumor selectively.
  - Monoclonal antibodies
  - Vaccines

Supportive Care

Follow-up after screening examinations is important, regardless of whether the screen was positive. Patients with NMSC and MM need to have life-long screening for development of second primary malignancies.

Chapter 57
· · · · · · · · · · · · ·

Stomach Cancer

Incidence
Gastric cancer is a problem worldwide. Incidence and mortality are increasing in some parts of the world, but they are decreasing in the United States. In the United States, there are about 13,000 deaths from gastric cancer each year. Overall, 5-year survival rates are 5% to 15% because gastric cancer is usually detected in advanced stages.

The highest incidence in the United States is seen among African Americans, Native Americans, and Hispanics. Males have a greater incidence than do females. Average age of onset is 50 to 70 years of age.

Etiology
Several conditions are strongly linked with the development of gastric cancer. Those risk factors with the highest correlation to gastric cancer are

- dietary intake of large amounts of nitrosamines and low amounts of fresh fruits and vegetables,
- infection with *Helicobacter pylori* (*H. pylori*),
- low socioeconomic class,
- prior gastric resection, and
- benign peptic ulcer disease.

Pathophysiology
More than 95% of gastric cancers are adenocarcinomas. Most cancers arise in the gastric antrum. About 10% invade the entire stomach, producing a rigid organ condition referred to as linitis plastica.

Progression of Disease

Gastric cancer is usually advanced at presentation. It can progress and metastasize by several routes:

- Direct extension into adjacent structures
- Local or distant nodal metastases
- Bloodstream metastases
- Intraperitoneal dissemination
- Distant metastatic sites: lung, adrenals, bone, and liver

Clinical Manifestations

Patients with early gastric cancer are typically asymptomatic or report vague complaints similar to other gastric ailments. Typical manifestations include

- reflux,
- abdominal pain,
- early satiety,
- indigestion,
- nausea and vomiting,
- weight loss,
- dysphagia, and
- anorexia.

Assessment

A complete history and physical examination can provide direction for further diagnostic study. Physical examination findings may include lymphadenopathy, hepatomegaly, or a palpable mass.

Diagnostic Studies

- CT is the most common study.
- Double-contrast upper gastrointestinal series
- Upper endoscopic gastroduodenoscopy (EGD)
- Direct biopsy and brushings
- Endoscopic gastroscopy

- Endoscopic ultrasound
- Bacteriology study for *H. pylori*
- Hematological profiles

Classification and Staging

Histological classification is of two types: intestinal and diffuse. The TNM designation is the common staging system. Lymph node metastases and number of positive nodes are strong predictors of prognosis.

Treatment

Localized tumors are treated with curative intent, using aggressive surgery alone or in combination with chemotherapy or radiotherapy. About 30% of patients are candidates for curative intent therapy.

Advanced tumors that are partially resectable, unresectable, or disseminated are treated with combination therapy using surgery and chemotherapy, with or without radiotherapy. In addition, palliative surgery may be performed to alleviate obstruction or restore intestinal continuity.

Surgery

Surgery should always be considered for gastric cancer, even with metastases. The choice of surgical procedure is based on location and extent of disease.

Types of surgical procedures for gastric cancer

- Total gastrectomy
  - For resectable lesions located in the body or midportion of the stomach
  - The entire stomach is removed, along with supporting mesentery and nodes.
  - The esophagus is anastomosed to the jejunum.
- Radical subtotal gastrectomy
  - For lesions in the middle and distal portions
  - Billroth I (gastroduodenostomy) is the choice

for debilitated individuals, because it is limited and not as extensive a resection as Billroth II.

- Billroth II (gastrojejunostomy) is used if the person can tolerate a more radical procedure and wider resection.
- Proximal subtotal gastrectomy
  - For tumor located in the proximal portion of the stomach or cardia
  - The stomach and distal esophagus are removed.
- Palliative surgical procedures
  - For relief of debilitating advanced symptoms, even if temporary
  - Resection to relieve obstruction, stop bleeding, or relieve pain

Potential complications following gastric surgery include

- pneumonia,
- hemorrhage,
- infection,
- reflux aspiration,
- anastomotic leak, and
- altered gastric emptying.

Potential typical postgastrectomy syndromes develop if a large amount of stomach has been removed. Not all patients will develop this problem. The classic sequela is termed *dumping syndrome* and may include any of the following symptoms:

- steatorrhea
- weight loss
- diarrhea
- nausea
- vitamin deficiency
- vomiting

Measures to minimize dumping syndrome

- Small, frequent feedings of low-carbohydrate, high-fat, high-protein foods

- Restriction of fluid for 30 minutes before and after meal
- Antispasmodics and antiperistaltics to reduce diarrhea
- Vitamin B12 deficiency replacement doses

Radiation Therapy

Gastric adenocarcinomas are generally radiosensitive. Radiation is often used with chemotherapy as adjuvant therapy following resection and to augment locoregional control of residual or advanced disease. Typical treatment is 4500 cGy over a 5-week period. Special attention must be given to the nutritional status of the patient. Side effects of radiation to gastric area are acute gastrointestinal symptoms, cramping, nausea, vomiting, and gastritis.

Chemotherapy

Adjuvant treatment is reserved for those diagnosed with advanced-stage disease. Combination drug therapy is superior to single agents, and combination chemotherapy regimens used are:

- FAM (5-fluorouracil [5-FU], doxorubicin, mitomycin-C)
- EAP (etoposide, doxorubicin, cisplatin)
- FAMTX (5-FU, doxorubicin, methotrexate)
- ELF (etoposide, leukovorin, 5-FU)
- 5-FU and cisplatin (most common regimen)

Supportive Care

Nutritional support is a nursing priority; however, nutrition therapy is often problematic because of either obstruction or dysfunction. Lack of gastric secretory function leads to enzyme and nutrient deficiencies needing replacement and monitoring. Pain, pulmonary complications, and dehydration can occur and need immediate attention.

Chapter 58

Testicular Cancer

Incidence
Testicular cancer accounts for approximately 1% of all cancers in males, and it is the most common solid tumor in men between ages 20 and 30. The incidence of testicular cancer in blacks and Asians is rare. This cancer is highly curable, especially if detected early.

Etiology
The cause of germ-cell tumors is unknown, but a history of testicular cancer; cryptorchidism; genetic, familial, and environmental factors; and hormones are considered risk factors. Young men should practice monthly testicular self-examination and report any lump or change in contour of the testicle.

Pathophysiology
Testicular tumors arise from germ tissue and are classified as either nonseminomatous germ-cell tumors or seminoma. Metastasis occurs either by extension or via lymphatics.

Clinical Manifestation
The most common presenting symptom of testis cancer is a painless swelling or enlargement of the testis. Other presenting symptoms include back pain (secondary to retroperitoneal adenopathy) and gynecomastia that can be unilateral or bilateral.

PART VI

Assessment
Physical examination includes a careful inspection of the scrotum. Transillumination of the

mass will diagnose a hydrocele. Lymph nodes are examined, especially the abdominal and supra-clavicular nodes.

Ultrasound is the test of choice for diagnosing testicular masses. Chest x-rays are valuable in determining whether a patient has gross metas-tases. CT scans provide information regarding retroperitoneal/pelvic disease.

Serum markers BCG and AFP are elevated in 85% of patients with disseminated nonseminomatous germ-cell tumors.

Classification and Staging

Several systems exist for the classification and staging of testicular cancer. The Royal Marsden Hospital Staging classification involves three sep-arate stages based on local and distant spread, whereas the Indiana University Staging System distinguishes minimal, moderate, and advanced disease.

- Patients with stage I (testis alone) and II (testis and retroperitoneal lymph nodes) seminoma-tous and nonseminomatous tumors should survive their disease.

- Patients with stage III disseminated disease with low serum markers or no evidence of pulmonary or mediastinal disease have a good prognosis. Patients with low tumor markers and/or limited disease have an excellent chance of cure.

- Patients with disseminated testicular cancer are associated with a greater than 90% cure rate with cisplatin-based combination chemotherapy.

Treatment

Treatment of nonseminoma germ cell tumors

- Retroperitoneal lymphadenectomy (RPLND) for stage I

- Adjuvant cisplatin-based chemotherapy after RPLND in stage II disease prevents relapse in nearly 100% of men.
- Disseminated disease treated with cisplatin-based chemotherapy: 30% require surgery (RPLND) after chemotherapy.

Treatment of seminomas

- Seminomas are uniquely sensitive to radiotherapy.
- With effective chemotherapy and radiotherapy, the overall cure rate for all stages is above 90%.
- 80% of seminomas present as clinical stage I disease.
- Stage I and stage II (nonbulky) disease is curable with external beam radiation.
- Chemotherapy is the primary treatment of bulky stage IIC and disseminated disease.

Supportive Care

Symptom management and nursing care focuses on the following:

- Fertility evaluation for men who wish to father a child in the future
- Anticipation of anxiety and threat to masculinity, sexual potency, and fertility
- Assurance of normal sexual functioning after unilateral orchiectomy
- Monitoring and management of side effects related to radiotherapy and chemotherapy
- Education, encouragement, and emotional support.

PART VI

Chapter 59

Vaginal Cancer

Incidence
Vaginal cancer is one of the rarest gynecological tumors, accounting for 1% to 2% of gynecological tumors. Peak incidence usually occurs in women between ages 50 and 70.

Etiology
Risk factors
- History of human papillomavirus (HPV)
- Herpes simplex virus type 2
- Long-term use of vaginal pessaries
- Radiation therapy
- Abdominal hysterectomy
- Lower educational level
- Lower socioeconomic status
- Age greater than 60 years
- Maternal use of diethylstilbestrol

Pathophysiology
Squamous carcinoma is most common cell type. There are two categories of vaginal tumors: vaginal intraepithelial neoplasia (VAIN) and invasive disease.

VAIN
- Divided into three subcategories: I, II, and III
- Usually seen in women treated for cervical intraepithelial neoplasia or after radiotherapy for cervical cancer

Invasive Vaginal Cancer
- Vaginal cancers occur most commonly on the posterior wall of the upper third of the vagina

and on the anterior wall of the lower third of the vagina.

- Tumor may spread along the vaginal wall into the cervix or vulva. Metastasis is typically to the lungs and supraclavicular nodes.

Clinical Manifestations

The most frequent symptom of vaginal cancer is abnormal bleeding that may occur after coitus. Other symptoms include foul-smelling discharge, dysuria, and urinary symptoms.

Assessment

Careful physical examination includes visual inspection of the mucosa and palpation of the vagina. Diagnostic measures typically used are

- Pap smear (for squamous cell, not adenocarcinoma),
- colposcopy,
- vaginal and cervical biopsies,
- chest x-ray,
- biochemical profile,
- intravenous pyelogram and barium enema, and
- cystoscopy.

Classification and Staging

The International Federation of Gynecology and Obstetrics (FIGO) system is commonly used. Staging is achieved by clinical staging. Overall 5-year survival is 50% to 65%. Survival for stage I is about 80%; for stage II, 65%; for stage III, 40%; and for stage IV, 15%.

PART VI

Treatment

Location of the lesion, its size, and whether it is single or multifocal determine the treatment selected.

VAIN

Women with VAIN I do not require any treatment. Women with VAIN II are treated with ablative therapy using laser or 5-fluorouracil (5-FU). VAIN III lesions should be excised because they are considered premalignant.

Invasive Disease

Radiation

Radiation is the most widely used treatment for vaginal cancer. For women with large stage I and stage II, III, or IV lesions, a combination of external radiation and brachytherapy is recommended. Vaginal fibrosis and scarring are major adverse effects of radiation. Desquamation of skin during therapy requires meticulous attention.

Surgery

For lesions in the upper vagina, a radical vaginectomy or radical hysterectomy may be done. Vaginal reconstruction occurs during vaginectomy. For larger lesions, a pelvic exenteration may be needed.

Chemotherapy

Few studies have been completed. 5-FU and cisplatin are the most common agents used. Mitomycin C has been used with radiation with some success.

Supportive Care

Education and support during aggressive therapies is critical. Constipation and blood in stool may occur with advanced disease. Laxatives are the first measures to use, but surgery may be necessary for obstruction. A rectovaginal fistula may occur and cause distressing fecal incontinence. Excellent wound management and meticulous hygiene will assist. The nurse may need to address changes in body image, alterations in sexuality, and coping mechanisms.

Chapter 60
....

Vulvar Cancer

Incidence
Vulvar cancer is a disease of elderly women and accounts for 3% to 5% of all gynecological cancers. Peak incidence occurs between ages 70 and 80, and it rarely occurs in women under age 40.

Vulvar cancer can be preceded by a preinvasive intraepithelial neoplasia of the vulvar tissue. *Vulvar intraepithelial neoplasia (VIN)* is a term used to note degrees of change. Thus, vulvar cancer is categorized as either

- preinvasive vulvar lesions (VIN I, II, III) or
- invasive vulvar cancer.

Etiology
The etiology of VIN and invasive vulvar cancer is unknown.

Risk Factors
- Human papillomavirus (type 16)
- *p53* tumor-suppressor gene
- Venereal warts
- Herpes simplex virus type 2 (HSV2)
- Multiple sexual partners
- Chronic vulvar disease
- History of smoking
- Previous malignancy of lower genital tract
- Advanced age (age 60 or older)

Pathophysiology
Vulvar cancer is a localized disease with well-defined margins. Ninety percent of cases are squamous cell cancers. The majority of vulvar

PART VI

cancers develop on the labia majora but can develop on the labia minora and clitoris.

Common routes of metastatic spread are direct extension and lymphatic dissemination to regional nodes (45% of cases). In advanced stages, vulvar cancer metastasizes to the urethra, vagina, rectum, and pubic bone.

Clinical Manifestations

VIN
- Approximately 50% of patients are asymptomatic. Other symptoms include vulvar pruritus, burning (vulvodynia), bleeding, discharge, or dysuria.
- A woman may delay seeking treatment, sometimes for 2 to 16 months.

Invasive Vulvar Cancer
- Twenty percent of patients are asymptomatic. Lesions are often detected during routine examinations. A less common finding is the presence of a mass or growth in the vulvar area.

Assessment
Diagnostic measures vary according to extent of disease.
- VIN
  - Inspection
  - Toluidine stain
  - Colposcopy
  - Biopsy
- Invasive vulvar cancer
  - Local excisional biopsy
  - Colposcopy
  - Pap smear
  - Complete examination of vulva, cervix, and vagina

The metastatic work-up includes

- chest x-ray,
- proctosigmoidoscopy,
- cystoscopy,
- barium enema,
- intravenous pyelogram, and
- biochemical profile.

Classification and Staging

Staging is according to the International Federation of Gynecology and Obstetrics (FIGO) system. Vulvar cancer has an overall 5-year survival rate of between 70% and 75% for all stages; survival is even higher for women with disease-negative nodes.

Treatment

Treatment varies according to the stage of disease and is predominantly surgical.

VIN

Treatment of VIN includes the following options:

- A wide local excision of the lesion with primary closure skin flaps or skin grafts is used most often.
- For multicentric disease, the treatment is a skinning vulvectomy. Vulvar skin is excised and a split-thickness skin graft is applied. This procedure requires prolonged bed rest for healing to occur.
- Local treatment with laser surgery, cryosurgery, or cautery may cause painful ulcerations that take 3 months to heal.
- Topical 5-fluorouracil (5-FU) cream in daily applications may be used to treat VIN. 5-FU may cause painful, slow-healing ulcers.

Invasive Vulvar Cancer

Surgery

- En bloc dissection of tumor, regional inguinal and femoral nodes, vulva, and sometimes pelvic nodes
- Nodal dissection also can be achieved through separate incisions in the groin, rather than by the en bloc approach.
- Early lesions: Stage I (less than 2 cm lesion with less than 5 mm of stromal invasion) are treated with a modified radical vulvectomy without groin dissection.
- Stage II and III lesions require more extensive surgery.
  - Radical vulvectomy
  - Bilateral inguinal-femoral lymphadenectomy
  - If needed, resection of surrounding organs: urethra, vagina, anus, rectum
- Stage IV disease
  - Pelvic exenteration may be required in addition to radical vulvectomy (if rectum or bladder is involved)
  - Radiotherapy may be used if the tumor is fixed or there are distant metastases.
- Possible complications after radical surgery
  - Wound breakdown, infection
  - Chronic leg edema
  - Recurrent cellulitis of leg
  - Deep venous thrombosis
  - Pulmonary embolism
  - Genital prolapse
  - Urinary stress incontinence

Radiation

Radiotherapy can be used in combination with surgery.

- Useful for those considered at high risk for re-currence

- Potential wound-healing problems with radiation

Chemotherapy

- Use of concurrent radiation and chemotherapy shows promise.
- 5-FU, cisplatin, and mitomycin C are the most common drugs used.

Supportive Therapy

Approximately 80% of recurrences will occur within the first 2 years after treatment. Those with fewer than three positive nodes have a low incidence of recurrence, whereas those with more than three nodes have a high incidence of recurrence.

Surgery is used to treat local recurrences, but recurrences may be treated with radiotherapy and surgery combined. Advanced tumors can be large, disfiguring, and painful. Nursing measures concentrate on patient education, prevention of pain, and infection.

Part VII

Appendices

Appendix 19A Oral Antineoplastic Agents

Drug and Disease Indications	Dose and Schedule	Side Effects: Acute or Delayed	Pharmacokinetics	Comments
Altretamine (Hexamethyl-melamine hexalene) Ovarian cancer	*Cap:* 50 mg and 100 mg clear Dose: 240–320 mg/m²/day	*Nadir:* 21–28 days Acute liver toxicity is dose-limiting; nausea and vomiting are dose-related Mild BMS (bone marrow suppression) Abdominal cramping Diarrhea Peripheral neuropathies Agitation, confusion	Variable absorption Rapid metabolism Urine excretion 90% in 72 hr	• Pyridoxine 50 mg/day may decrease neuropathy. • Take with food, prophylactic antiemetics. • May worsen vincristine-related peripheral neuropathy.
Busulfan (Myleran) Leukemia	*Tab:* 2 mg white Dose: 4–12 mg/day for several weeks	*Nadir:* 10–30 days delayed marrow recovery Potentially teratogenic Pulmonary fibrosis with long-term use Dermatologic hyperpigmentation Gynecomastia Amenorrhea	Well absorbed Extensive hepatic metabolism to inactive compounds Renal excretion	• Bone marrow recovery may be delayed; therefore caution is advised with long-term use. Hydration and allopurinol may be indicated to prevent hyperuricemia. Total cumulative dose: 600 mg. • Long-term daily administration is not recommended due to the risk of second malignancies with chronic alkylating agents.
Capecitabine (Xeloda) Metastatic breast cancer	*Tab:* 150 mg light peach, 500 mg peach 2500 mg/m²/day × 14 days q 21 days swallow with	Mild BMS Dose-limiting toxicity is diarrhea Hand-foot syndrome, dermatitis, fatigue, anorexia, nausea, stomatitis	Metabolized to 5-FU; excreted in urine Hepatic metabolism to active compound	• Administer in two oral doses, 12 hours apart, 30 minutes after a meal • Monitor coagulation profile in patients also taking coumarin

Drug (Indications)	Dose	Pharmacokinetics	Nursing Considerations
Chlorambucil (Leukeran) Leukemia Hodgkin's disease	*Tab:* 2 mg white *Dose:* 4–8 mg/m²/day × 3–6 wk 16 mg/m²/wk q 4 wk *Nadir:* 7–10 days Severe BMS Slight nausea and vomiting Occasional dermatitis Abnormal liver function Pulmonary fibrosis with prolonged use Second malignancy Sterility	Renal excretion of 50% of unchanged drug	• Good oral absorption. • Concomitant barbiturate administration may enhance toxicity. Marrow suppression may be prolonged.
Cyclophosphamide (Cytoxan) Breast cancer Multiple myeloma Small cell lung cancer Malignant lymphomas Leukemias	water only; take with food *Tab:* 25–50 mg *Dose:* 1–5 mg/kg/day 60–120 mg/m² Adjust dose in presence of renal dysfunction *Nadir:* 7–14 days Bone marrow suppression (BMS) Anorexia, nausea, and vomiting Alopecia Hemorrhagic cystitis gross or microscopic hematuria Amenorrhea Sterility	Activated in the liver Oral absorption in 1 hr 30% of drug excreted unchanged in urine	• Vigorous hydration (3 L/day). • Encourage frequent voiding to prevent hemorrhagic cystitis (a sterile inflammation of the urinary bladder). If patient complains of burning on urination or bladder incontinence, urinalysis may reveal occult blood. Control by withdrawal of the drug and hydration. • May take pills in divided doses early in the day and with meals or all at one time. Better tolerated with cold foods. • Barbiturates and other inducers of hepatic microsomal enzymes may enhance toxicity, e.g., cimetidine. Allopurinol may enhance BMS.

PART VII

Appendix 19A Oral Antineoplastic Agents (continued)

Drug and Disease Indications	Dose and Schedule	Side Effects: Acute or Delayed	Pharmacokinetics	Comments
Hydroxyurea (Hydrea) Chronic myelocytic leukemia Melanoma Head and neck cancer	*Cap:* 500 mg *Dose:* 80 mg/kg/day every third day 750–1000 mg/m²/day × 5 Decrease dose in presence of renal dysfunction Store in tight container in a cool environment	*Nadir:* 13–17 days Acute nausea and vomiting Chronic and severe anemia Neurological seizures and hallucinations Dermatitis Dysuria Azotemia	Well absorbed Hepatic metabolism Renal excretion of 80% of compound in 12 hr Crosses into CSF	• Concomitant radiation and/or 5-fluorouracil (5-FU) may enhance neurotoxicity. • Dysuria and renal impairment may occur. • Consider pretreatment with allopurinol.
Gleevec Chronic myeloid leukemia (CML)	*Dose:* 400 mg/day for patients in chronic phase CML; 600 mg/day for patients in accelerated phase or blast crisis Administer once daily with a meal and a large glass of water.	Neutropenia and thrombocytopenia are dose dependent. Hepatotoxicity has been reported. Nausea, vomiting, edema, and muscle cramps have been reported. Fluid retention is dose related Hepatotoxicity may occur.	Inhibits proliferation and induces apoptosis of bcr-abl positive cell lines. It is a protein tyrosine kinase inhibitor Well absorbed within 2–4 hours of administration. Elimination half life is 18–40 hours	• Drugs like ketoconazole or erythromycin may increase plasma concentrations of Gleevec. • Dexamethasone, phenobarbital, or St. John's Wort may reduce concentration of Gleevec.
Lomustine (CCNU) Brain cancer Lymphomas	*Cap:* 100 mg green/green, 40 mg green/white, 10 mg white	*Nadir:* 28–42 days Severe cumulative BMS Nausea and vomiting 4–6 hr after dosing	Absorbed rapidly (<60 min) Hepatic metabolism	• Dispense one dose at a time to prevent accidental overdose. • Take on an empty stomach just before bedtime.

Drug	Dose	Toxicity	Pharmacokinetics	Comments
L-phenylanine mustard (Melphalan, Alkeran) Multiple myeloma Ovarian cancer	*Dose:* 100–130 mg/m² q 6–8 wk	Anorexia Alopecia Stomatitis Hepatotoxicity	Renal excretion of 50% in 24 hr and 75% in 96 hr Crosses into CSF	• Pretreat with aggressive antiemetics. • Protect pills from heat and humidity.
	Tab: 2 mg white *Dose:* 0.1–0.15 mg/kg/day × 2–3 wk Reduce dose with hepatic or renal impairment	*Nadir:* 10–18 days Nausea and vomiting usually mild Dermatitis Pulmonary fibrosis Long-term therapy can result in acute leukemia	Hepatic metabolism Renal excretion 20%–35% (10% unchanged) 20%–50% excreted in feces within 6 days	• Protect pills from sunlight. • Take on an empty stomach. • BMS may be cumulative in older patients. • Leukemogenic.
6-Mercaptopurine (6-MP) Leukemia	*Tab:* 50 mg off-white *Dose:* 80–100 mg/m²/day Titrate dose based on blood counts Reduce dose in presence of hepatic or renal dysfunction	*Nadir:* 10–14 days Nausea, vomiting Mucositis Diarrhea Drug fever Intrahepatic cholestasis Pulmonary toxicity with prolonged use	Incomplete oral absorption Hepatic inactivation Renal excretion 10% unchanged in 24 hr	• Protect pills from light. • Administer as single dose on an empty stomach. • Increased toxicity with allopurinol (reduce dose by one-third to one-fourth of the original dose). • Administer with caution to patients on sodium warfarin (Coumadin). • Monitor liver function tests.
Methotrexate Squamous cell carcinoma Lung cancer	*Tab:* 2.5 mg yellow *Dose:* 2.5–10 mg/day PO or 15–30 mg/day PO × 5 days q 1–3 wk	*Nadir:* 7–10 days Nausea and anorexia can occur; stomatitis and ulcerations can occur and are dose-limiting.	Serum half-life is 2–4 hr Excreted by the kidneys	• Dose is reduced with renal impairment; dosing on an empty stomach may enhance bioavailability. Excretion may be impaired in patients with simultaneous administration of weak acids such as salicylates or vitamin C; oral dosing is generally well tolerated. • Avoid administration of methotrexate with ketoprotein or probenecid because toxicity of methotrexate may be enhanced.

Appendix 19A Oral Antineoplastic Agents (continued)

Drug and Disease

Indications	Dose and Schedule	Side Effects: Acute or Delayed	Pharmacokinetics	Comments
Procarbazine (Matulane) Hodgkin's disease	*Cap:* 50 mg *Dose:* 100 mg/m²/day × 14 days q 4 wk; reduce dose in presence of hepatic or renal dysfunction	*Nadir:* 4 wk BMS, nausea, vomiting, and diarrhea gradually subside; flulike syndrome, paresthesias, neuropathies, dizziness, and ataxia	Well absorbed from the gastrointestinal tract Metabolized in the liver with a biological half-life of about 1 hr 70% of the drug is eliminated by 24 hr in the urine; 5% appears as unchanged drug	• Drug and food interactions can occur. • Central nervous system (CNS) depression can occur with concomitant administration of procarbazine and CNS depressants. • Hypertensive crisis can occur when procarbazine is administered with certain antidepressants (tricyclics and monoamine oxidase inhibitors) and tyramine-rich foods. • Severe nausea and vomiting can occur if taken with ethanol, mixed drinks, and beer.
Temozolomide (Temodar) Astrocytoma	*Cap:* 5 mg green, 20 mg brown, 100 mg blue, 250 mg black *Dose:* 150 mg/m²/day × 5 days q mo Dose escalation based on nadir counts	*Nadir:* Platelets by day 26, neutrophils by day 28 BMS is dose-limiting toxicity Nausea, vomiting, fatigue, and headache can be severe in 10% of cases	Rapidly absorbed with a mean elimination half-life of 1.8 hr Eliminated via the kidneys	• Take on an empty stomach at night with glass of water. • Capsules should not be opened or chewed.
6-Thioguanine Leukemia	*Tab:* 40 mg green/yellow *Dose:* 80–100 mg/m²	*Nadir:* 7–28 days Stomatitis	Variable, incomplete absorption	• Administer on an empty stomach. • Does not require dose reduction when used in con-

VP-16	Reduce dose if stomatitis occurs	Diarrhea	Hepatic metabolism	junction with allopurinol.
(etoposide, VePesid)		Hepatotoxicity	Renal excretion	•Nausea is mild though can be more severe with oral route than with IV route.
Lung cancer	*Cap:* 50 mg pink	*Nadir:* 7-14 days (white blood cell count)	Renal and hepatic metabolism	
Testicular cancer	*Dose:* 2 × the IV dose or	Nausea and vomiting: 9-16 days (platelets)	Incomplete and variable absorption	
	100-200 mg/m²/day × 3-5	Alopecia		
	days q 3-4 wk	BMS is dose limiting		

Adapted and revised from Goodman M: Delivery of cancer chemotherapy, in Baird S, McCorkle R, Grant M (eds): Cancer Nursing: A Comprehensive Textbook. Philadelphia, Saunders, 1991, p 311.

Appendix 19B Intravenous Antineoplastic Agents

Dosage and Efficacy	Mechanism of Action and Metabolism	Administration Precautions	Side Effects
	BLEOMYCIN (Blenoxane)		
Dosage: • May be given IM, SQ, IV, intratumoral, intra-arterial. • 10–20 U/m² once or twice a week • Intrapleural/pericardial sclerosing dose: 50–60 U/m² in 50–100 mL NS or D5W; not to exceed 40 U/m² in geriatric population *Efficacy:* • Cervical cancer • Head and neck cancer • Penis, skin, and testicular cancer • Hodgkin's and non-Hodgkin's lymphoma • Kaposi's sarcoma	*Mechanism of action:* • Cell-cycle phase specific for G_2 and M phase. Binds to DNA. • Inhibits cell progression out of G_2, resulting in cellular synchronization for subsequent drug therapy. *Metabolism:* • t ½ = 20 min • Renal elimination	*Administration precautions:* • Administer with caution to patients with significant pulmonary or renal disease. Prior cisplatin therapy may reduce bleomycin clearance, increasing plasma half-life and toxicity. • Test dose: Bleomycin is associated with HSR and a test dose of 2 U IV in 50 mL D5W over 15 min followed by observation. Observe for anaphylactic reaction for 1–2 hours posttest dose. • Lymphoma patients are more at risk for HSR and should be tested for the first two doses.	*Side effects:* • Lifetime cumulative dose is 400 U. • 25% dose reduction for creatinine clearance of 30–50 mL/min • 50% dose reduction for creatinine clearance of 20–30 mL/min • Fever occurs in approximately 50% of patients. Premedicate with acetaminophen 1 g and diphenhydramine 50 mg. (Repeat 6 hr later.) • Dermatological reactions such as hyperpigmentation, hyperkeratosis, and erythema on palms and fingers; urticaria, rash, mucositis, and alopecia • Anorexia and mild nausea • Interstitial pneumonitis and pulmonary fibrosis occur more commonly in patients who also have mediastinal radiation, are elderly, and receive higher cumulative doses.

CARBOPLATIN (Paraplatin)

Dosage:

- IV: 360 mg/m² q 4 wk
- Higher doses are given in pretransplant protocols and intraperitoneally or intraarterially.
- Dose calculations are most therapeutically based on the desired serum concentration (AUC), renal status, and whether or not the patient has been previously treated with chemotherapy (Calvert Method).
- Note that doses calculated according to the Calvert formula are total mg, not mg/m² (see text).

Efficacy:

- Ovarian carcinoma
- Testicular cancer
- Head and neck cancer
- Cervical cancer
- Lung cancer

Mechanism of action:

- Maximal cytotoxicity occurs when cells are in the S-phase although cell kill by intrastrand DNA cross-linkage occurs throughout G_1, S, and G_2 phases of the cell cycle.

Metabolism:

- $t\frac{1}{2} = 2.5$ hr
- 60% eliminated unchanged in the urine
- Major routes of elimination are glomerular filtration and tubular secretion.

Administration precautions:

- Available as lyophilized (powdered) form to distinguish it from cisplatin, which is only available in aqueous solution.
- Usually administered over 15-30 min in 500 mL of NS or D5W, without further hydration.
- May also be administered as a continuous 24-hr or longer infusion.
- Forms a precipitate when in contact with aluminum, causing loss of antitumor potency.
- Injection site irritation and erythema can occur with infiltration but no ulceration or necrosis.
- Physically compatible with ondansetron.

Side effects:

- DLT: myelosuppression, particularly thrombocytopenia. Nadir occurs at 2-3 wk.
- Nausea and vomiting are mild and rarely last beyond 24 hours.
- Ototoxicity and neurotoxicity (paresthesias) are uncommon.
- Alopecia, mucositis, and abnormal liver functions have been reported.
- Nephrotoxicity occurs but is less common than with cisplatin.

CARMUSTINE (BiCNU)

Dosage:

- IV: 150-200 mg/m² q 6 wk
- Higher doses have been used in pretransplant protocols.

Mechanism of action:

- Inhibits enzymatic reactions involved in DNA synthesis
- Inhibits DNA repair

Administration precautions:

- Soluble in water and absolute alcohol.
- Protect from light.
- Administer in 100-500 mL D5W or NS as a

Side effects:

- DLT: Leukopenia and thrombocytopenia occur 3-5 wk after treatment, recovery at 8 wk.
- Myelosuppression may be cumulative.

Appendix 19B Intravenous Antineoplastic Agents (continued)

Dosage and Efficacy	Mechanism of Action and Metabolism	Administration Precautions	Side Effects
Efficacy: • Brain tumors • Multiple myeloma • Hodgkin's disease • Non-Hodgkin's lymphoma • Melanoma	• Acts predominantly during late G and early S phase • Readily crosses the blood-brain barrier *Metabolism:* • Metabolized by the liver • 80% eliminated via the kidneys • t ½ = 15-20 min	• 1- to 2-hr infusion. • Infusion may burn as it goes in and should be monitored closely. • Heat provides symptomatic relief. • Slowing the infusion rate also eases vein discomfort. • Hypotension can occur if the infusion is given rapidly. • Facial flushing and dizziness occur infrequently. • Compatible with ondansetron. • Incompatible with polyvinylchloride infusion bags and with sodium bicarbonate. • Avoid contact with skin; a brown stain may result.	• Nausea and vomiting are common and require aggressive antiemetic therapy. • Pulmonary fibrosis has been reported and generally presents as a dry cough and dyspnea. • Alopecia is common. • Elevation of LFTs and azotemia can occur with higher doses. Cimetidine has been shown to potentiate carmustine toxicity.

CISPLATIN (Platinol) AQUEOUS SOLUTION

Dosage: • IV: 20-40 mg/m² day × 3-5 days q 3-4 wk • 20-120 mg/m² single dose q 3-4 wk • IP: 100-270 mg/m² in 2 L of warmed NS. In-	*Mechanism of action:* • Binds to DNA affecting DNA replication • Forms DNA protein cross-links • Interacts with cellular glutathione	*Administration precautions:* • Dose reductions: 25% dose reduction for patients with creatinine clearance of 30-50 mL/min and a 50% dose reduction for pa-	*Side effects:* • Concomitant administration of probenecid enhances cisplatin renal toxicity. • Monitor patient for HSR: tachycardia, wheez-

fuse via gravity over 10 min. Allow 4-hr dwell time.

Efficacy:
- Bladder
- Ovarian
- Testicular carcinoma
- Non-small cell lung cancer
- Head and neck cancer

Metabolism:
- 90% bound to plasma proteins
- 20%–45% eliminated unchanged via kidney
- $t\frac{1}{2} = 60$-90 hr
- 10% eliminated in bile

tients with creatinine clearance <30 mL/min
- Administer after appropriate hydration (1-2 L with mannitol).
- Maintain urinary output (125 mL/hr). Mixing cisplatin in 0.9% NaCl maintains drug stability.
- Cisplatin may react with aluminum resulting in loss of cisplatin potency.
- Physically compatible with ondansetron.
- Sodium thiosulfate and mesna directly inactivate cisplatin.
- Administer with caution in patients receiving other potentially nephrotoxic drugs (aminoglycosides).

ing, hypotension, and facial edema.
- Acute and delayed nausea and vomiting are preventable with aggressive antiemetics including 5 HT3 receptor antagonists, dexamethasone, and metoclopramide.
- High frequency hearing loss may occur in up to 30% of patients.
- Tinnitis, vestibular dysfunction, and ototoxicity occur infrequently and are preventable with adequate hydration and mannitol diuresis.
- Peripheral neuropathy including numbness, tingling, and sensory loss occurs in arms and legs with long-term administration.
- Hypomagnesemia is seen with high dose (>200 mg/m^2) and is preventable with oral and IV supplements.
- Hemolytic anemia is seen with higher doses and responds to recombinant erythropoietin.

CYCLOPHOSPHAMIDE (Cytoxan)

Dosage:
- PO: 50-200 mg/m^2 PO each day × 14 days q 28 days

Mechanism of action:
- Activated by hepatic microsomal enzymes; prevents cell division by cross-linking DNA

Administration precautions:
- When doses >1000 mg are given, patients should receive hydration of 500-1000 mL NS.

Side effects:
- Hemorrhagic cystitis occurs rarely with conventional doses.

Appendix 19B Intravenous Antineoplastic Agents (continued)

Dosage and Efficacy	Mechanism of Action and Metabolism	Administration Precautions	Side Effects
• IV: 500 mg–1.5 g/m² IV q 3 wk or 60 mg/kg IV × 2 days prior to BMT *Efficacy:* • Breast • Ovary • Leukemias • Lymphomas • Multiple myeloma • Lung cancer	strands • Non-cell-cycle phase specific *Metabolism:* • t ½ = 3–10 hr • Metabolized in the liver • Excreted in the kidney (15% unchanged) • 33% of drug is excreted unchanged in the stool	• Administer IV dose slowly to prevent nasal congestion, headache, and dizziness. • Encourage fluid intake of 3 L/day while taking cyclophosphamide. • When taking oral doses, encourage patient to take all pills before 5 P.M. to minimize bladder contact with toxic metabolites. • Phenytoin and chloral hydrate may enhance the conversion of cyclophosphamide to toxic metabolites, thereby increasing toxicity.	• Hydration and mesna are indicated with high-dose and pretransplant therapy. • SIADH can occur with high-dose cyclophosphamide. • Nausea and vomiting are preventable with aggressive antiemetic therapy. • Alopecia is common. Metallic taste occurs during injection and when taken orally. Encourage the patient to chew gum, peppermint, or lemon candy. • Myelosuppression (leukopenia) is dose-limiting. • Amenorrhea and reversible oligospermia occur and are dose dependent. • Cyclophosphamide 1 mg/mL is compatible with doxorubicin, cisplatin, mesna, and other drugs. • Blurring of vision has been reported. • Cardiac toxicity can occur with high-dose therapy, especially if given with radiation to the chest area.

CYTARABINE (Cytosar; ARA-C, Cytosine Arabinoside)

Dosage:
- IV: 5-10 day CI (continuous infusion) of 100-200 mg/m²
- Intrathecal: 5-70 mg/m² 1-3×/week
- Subcutaneous: 1 mg/kg 1-2×/week or 100 mg bid × 5 days q 28 days

Efficacy:
- Acute leukemia
- Myeloid leukemia
- Acute nonlymphocytic leukemia
- Meningeal leukemia

Mechanism of action:
- Inhibits DNA polymerase causing DNA chain elongation and arrest
- Cell-cycle phase specific for the S phase
- Antimetabolite

Metabolism:
- Metabolized in the liver
- At 24 hr, 90% of the drug is eliminated in the urine
- t½ = 2-3 hr

Administration precautions:
- Given IV push or IV infusion over 30 min
- 5- to 10-day continuous infusions may be optimal for antitumor cytotoxicity because of the S-phase specificity.
- For intrathecal use, mix drug with lactated Ringer's solution or NS without preservatives.
- Rotate sites for SQ injections.

Side effects:
- Myelosuppression is the DLT. Nadir at 5-7 days, recovery in 2-3 wk.
- Anemia is common.
- Nausea, vomiting, anorexia, metallic taste, stomatitis, and diarrhea are reported.
- Minimal alopecia
- Skin erythema can occur. Arthralgias and myalgias occur.
- After intrathecal use, patients may experience nausea, vomiting, fever, and headache.
- Ocular toxicity: excessive tearing, photophobia, and blurred vision.
- High-dose therapy can lead to CNS toxicity: lethargy, confusion, ataxia.
- Cytarabine may decrease the cellular uptake of methotrexate.
- Compatible with vincristine, prednisolone, sodium phosphate, and ondansetron.
- Physical changes are noted with methotrexate and 5-FU and heparin.
- Compatible with vancomycin for 4-8 hr.

Appendix 19B Intravenous Antineoplastic Agents (continued)

Dosage and Efficacy	Mechanism of Action and Metabolism	Administration Precautions	Side Effects
		DACARBAZINE (DTIC)	
Dosage: • 375 mg/m² q 3-4 wk or • 150-250 mg/m²/qd × 5 days q 3-4 wk or • 850 mg/m² on day 1 q 3-4 wk *Efficacy:* • Malignant melanoma • Soft tissue sarcomas • Hodgkin's disease	*Mechanism of action:* • Causes cross-linkage and breaks in DNA strands. • Inhibits RNA and DNA synthesis. • Cell-cycle phase nonspecific, but has more activity in late G_2. *Metabolism:* • Activated by liver microsomes • Excreted renally • $t\frac{1}{2} = 35$ min	*Administration precautions:* • Reconstitute with D5W or saline. • Solution can be painful and should be administered slowly in 250-500 mL of solution over 30-60 min. Moist heat along the vein eases pain. • Stable for 8 hr at room temperature, 72 hr if refrigerated. • Drug should be protected from light. • May turn to a pinkish color if exposed to light. • HSR can occur; hypotension occurs with high-dose therapy.	*Side effects:* • DLI: moderate degree of myelosuppression. • Nadir occurs at 21-25 days. • Anemia can occur. • Severe nausea and vomiting can occur. • Aggressive pretreatment with antiemetic therapy is needed. Nausea and vomiting lessen by day 3-4 of treatment. • Hepatotoxic; monitor liver functions • Flulike syndrome may occur with fever, myalgia, and malaise at about 7 days, lasting 1-3 wk. • Photosensitivity can occur; protect skin from sunlight.
		DACTINOMYCIN (Actinomycin D; ACT-D, Cosmegen)	
Dosage: • 10-15 µ/kg/day × 5 days q 3-4 wk or	*Mechanisms of action:* • Binds between purine-pyrimidine base pairs in DNA.	*Administration precautions:* • Reconstitute with preservative-free sterile water for injection. Preserved diluent may	*Side effects:* • DLI: myelosuppression occurs within 7-10 days of dosing.

- 2.4 mg/m^2 in divided doses over 1 wk

or

- 2 mg/m^2 IV q 3-4 wk

Efficacy:
- Wilms' tumor
- Embryonal rhabdomyosarcoma
- Choriocarcinoma
- Malignant melanoma
- Hodgkin's and non-Hodgkin's lymphoma

- Inhibits the synthesis of DNA-dependent RNA and messenger RNA.
- Action is cell-cycle nonspecific but is more active during G$_1$ and in cells that are cycling.

Metabolism:
Excreted unchanged in bile and urine

cause precipitation. Use drug as soon as possible.
- Monitor liver functions; dose reductions may be necessary.
- Use extreme caution during administration.
- Dactinomycin is a severe vesicant.
- Dactinomycin is compatible with ondansetron.
- When calculating dose, double-check the order since the drug is ordered both as μg/kg and mg/m^2.

- Nadir may be delayed, occurring at 3 wk.
- Due to its immunosuppressive effects, avoid administering dactinomycin to patients who have an active viral infection.
- Nausea and vomiting can be severe. Aggressive pretreatment with antiemetics is appropriate.
- Mucositis and diarrhea can be severe; institute preventive oral hygiene regimen.
- Alopecia occurs commonly.
- Erythema, hyperpigmentation, and an acne-like rash occur commonly.
- Dactinomycin can cause a radiation recall reaction.
- Hepatic venoocclusive toxicity manifested as elevated SGOT and bilirubin can occur.

DAUNORUBICIN (daunomycin, Cerubidine)

Dosage:
- 30-60 mg/m^2 daily × 3-5 days q 3-4 wk

Efficacy:
- ALL
- AML

Mechanism of action:
- Intercalates DNA, thereby blocking DNA, RNA and protein synthesis. It is an anthracycline antitumor antibiotic.

Administration precautions:
- 20-mg vial is reconstituted with 4 mL of sterile water = 5 mg/mL.
- QS to 15-20 mL of NS
- Stable for 24 hr at room temperature and 48 hr under refrigeration.

Side effects:
- DLT: myelosuppression.
- WBC nadir occurs at 7-14 days; recovery at 3 wk. Thrombocytopenia and anemia occur.
- Stomatitis occurs, but is mild.

396

Appendix 19B Intravenous Antineoplastic Agents (continued)

Dosage and Efficacy	Mechanism of Action and Metabolism	Administration Precautions	Side Effects
• Acute monocytic leukemia • Acute nonlymphocytic leukemia	*Metabolism:* • Metabolized in the liver • About 40% of the drug is eliminated via the bile • 20%–25% is eliminated via the urine • t½ = 20–25 hr	• Incompatible with heparin, 5-FU, and dexamethasone. • Compatible with ondansetron. • CAUTION: Because the solution is red, as is doxorubicin and with a similar sounding name, the vial should be double-checked against the order. • Urine will be pink to red for 12–24 hr after administration. • Daunorubicin is a severe vesicant. Extreme caution should be used in administration of this drug. • Administer via the side arm of a freely running IV or by the two-syringe technique.	• Diarrhea occurs infrequently. • Nausea and vomiting occur 1–5 hr after dosing but is prevented with aggressive antiemetic therapy. • Alopecia is abrupt and involves all body hair. • Hyperpigmentation of the nails occurs. Urticaria and a generalized rash have been reported. • Monitor liver functions. If elevated LFTs are noted, dose reduction is indicated. • Cardiac toxicity can occur. Dose is limited to 500–600 mg/m². • Manifestation of CHF is characterized by dyspnea on exertion, fatigue, and arrhythmias.

DOCETAXEL (Taxotere)

Dosage: • 80–100 mg/m² q 3 wk as a 1-hour infusion	*Mechanism of action:* • Antimicrotubule agent—a mitotic spindle poison. Enhances microtubule assembly and	*Administration precautions:* • Docetaxel solution contains 2 mg (40 mg/mL) of docetaxel in polysorbate/tween	*Side effects:* • The DLT for docetaxel is neutropenia and thrombocytopenia.

Efficacy:
- Ovarian cancer
- Breast cancer
- Non-small cell lung cancer

inhibits the depolymerization of tubulin. This process leads to increased bundles of microtubules in the cell. The cell is then unable to divide.

Metabolism:
- Metabolized in the liver, excreted in the feces, and minimally excreted in the urine.
- $t\frac{1}{2}$ = 11 hr

80. Refrigerated vial sits at room temperature for 5 min. Once mixed with solvent the solution contains 10 mg/mL. The appropriate amount of docetaxel is mixed with D5W in a concentration <1 mg/mL. Once diluted, docetaxel is stable for 8 hr at room temperature.
- Avoid infiltration: The drug is an irritant, but can cause tissue damage depending on the concentration.
- Apply cold to site, not heat.
- Monitor liver functions carefully; dose adjustments are appropriate if LFTs are elevated 2.5 × normal.

- All patients receive dexamethasone 8 mg PO bid × 5 days starting 1 day prior to docetaxel.
- Diphenhydramine 50 mg is also given 30 min prior to prevent hypersensitivity reactions.
- If mild HSR occurs with flushing, skin reactions, or pruritus, the infusion rate is slowed with observation. If the patient experiences rash, flushing, mild dyspnea, or chest discomfort, the infusion is stopped and the patient is treated with IV diphenhydramine and dexamethasone. The infusion may be resumed after symptoms abate.
- If severe symptoms such as generalized urticaria, angioedema, or hypotension occur, the infusion is stopped and the patient is treated with antihistamine, steroid, and if necessary epinephrine or bronchodilators. The patient may still receive the docetaxel depending on the severity of the response. If the patient reacts a second time the patient probably should not receive the drug again.
- Nausea and vomiting are minimal.
- Alopecia occurs within 3 wk of the first treatment.

Dosage and Efficacy	Mechanism of Action and Metabolism	Administration Precautions	Side Effects
			• Nail separation may occur.
			• Drug-associated fluid retention or edema including pleural effusions, ascites, and peripheral edema occur and may be managed with a diuretic, which may or may not be helpful.

DOXORUBICIN (Adriamycin, Rubex)

Dosage:	*Mechanism of action:*	*Administration precautions:*	*Side effects:*
• 60-75 mg/m² as bolus or as a continuous infusion over 3-4 days q 3-4 wk. Higher doses are used in dose-intensive regimens.	• Binds directly to DNA base pairs and inhibits DNA, RNA, and protein synthesis. Antitumor antibiotic. Cell-cycle specific for the S-phase.	• Available in liquid and lyophilized form.	• DLI: Myelosuppression, especially leukopenia. Nadir occurs at 10-14 days. Recovery is swift at 3 wk.
• Doxorubicin may also be given intraarterially, intrapleurally, and by bladder instillation.	*Metabolism:*	• Reconstitute with sterile water for injection, D5W, NS to form a solution of 2 mg/mL.	• Cardiac toxicity can occur. Dose is limited to 450-550 mg/m². Doxorubicin causes damage to the myocyte of the heart, causing various degrees of damage, but manifests as CHF as the heart begins to function less efficiently as a pump.
Efficacy:	• Extensively metabolized by the liver	• Stable for 35 days at room temperature.	
• Acute nonlymphocytic leukemia	• 40%-50% of the drug is eliminated in the bile.	• Incompatible with heparin, dexamethasone, 5-FU, furosemide, aminophylline.	
• Acute lymphocytic leukemia	• 5% is eliminated in the urine.	• Compatible with cyclophosphamide, cisplatin, dacarbazine, droperidol, vinblastine, vincristine, and ondansetron.	• MUGA scans are done periodically to monitor left ventricular function. Early symptoms of CHF include tachycardia, dyspnea on exertion, arrhythmias, and EKG changes.
• Wilms' tumor	• t ½ = 18-30 hr	• Doxorubicin turns the urine a reddish orange for 8-10 hr after administration.	
• Neuroblastoma		• Since doxorubicin is metabolized and eliminated by the liver, liver function tests are	
• Soft tissue sarcoma			
• Breast cancer			

- Hepatocellular carcinoma
- Ovarian carcinoma

monitored frequently. Elevation in bilirubin to 1.2-3 mg/dL warrants a 50% dose reduction; bilirubin of 3 mg/dL calls for a 75% dose reduction.
- Administer with extreme caution. Doxorubicin is a severe vesicant. It will cause tissue damage, ulceration, and necrosis if infiltrated. Inject through the side arm of a freely running and well-established IV or by using the two-syringe technique.
- CAUTION: It has a similar name and color to daunorubicin. Check the drug order against the vial to ensure the right dose of the right drug.

- Alopecia occurs predictably and is dose dependent. Doses greater than 50 mg are associated with moderate to severe loss. Doses of 90-100 mg cause hair loss in 2.5 wk.
- Stomatitis is dose-limiting and can be more severe with continuous infusions. Continuous infusions are only given through central lines, never through peripheral lines.
- Nail bed changes occur and include hyperpigmentation especially in blacks and in individuals of Mediterranean descent.

DOXORUBICIN HYDROCHLORIDE LIPOSOME INJECTION (Doxil)

Mechanism of action:
- Anti-tumor antibiotic binds directly to DNA
- Inhibits DNA and RNA synthesis
- Drug is encapsulated in stealth liposomes to prolong circulation time

Metabolism:
- Slower clearance from body than doxorubicin
- t½ = 55 hr

Administration precautions:
- Dilute in 250 mL 5% dextrose USP.
- Drug is an irritant.

Side effects:
- Acute infusion reaction may occur with flushing, shortness of breath, facial swelling, headache, chills, back pain, chest and throat tightness, and/or hypotension. Stop infusion. Restart if symptoms abate.
- Hand-foot syndrome may require dose reduction.

Dosage:
- 20 mg/m² over 30 min q 3 wk

Efficacy:
- AIDS
- Kaposi's sarcoma

Appendix 19B Intravenous Antineoplastic Agents (contined)

Dosage and Efficacy	Mechanism of Action and Metabolism	Administration Precautions	Side Effects
			• Stomatitis may occur.
			• BMS is dose limiting.
			• Cardiac toxicity may occur.
			• Less incidence of alopecia compared to doxorubicin.

EPIRUBICIN (Ellence)

Dosage and Efficacy	Mechanism of Action and Metabolism	Administration Precautions	Side Effects
Dosage: • 100–120 mg/m^2 IV every 3–4 weeks as adjuvant therapy in axillary node positive breast cancer • Divided dose may be given day 1 and 8 or over 2–3 days or IV every week. *Efficacy:* • Breast cancer	*Mechanism of action:* • Acts on DNA base pairs inhibiting nucleic acid and protein synthesis. Cleavage of DNA by topoisomerase II causes cell death. *Metabolism:* • T½ is approximately 30–40 hours. • Extensively metabolized by the liver. • Elimination occurs through the bile and urine.	*Administration precautions:* • Drug is provided in a ready to use solution (50 mg/25 ml and 200 mg/100 ml) • Use within 24 hours of penetration of rubber stopper. • Store in refrigerator. • Drug is a vesicant-administer via slow IVP into the side port of a freely flowing IV infusion as per protocol. • Drug dosage should be modified if the patient has renal or hepatic dysfunction. • Drug should not be administered with cimetidine as it increases drug AUC by 50%.	*Side effects:* • DLI: Myelosuppression with nadir at 10–14 days after drug dose. Thrombocytopenia and anemia may be severe. • Nausea and vomiting are preventable with antiemetics. • Anorexia, diarrhea, and mucositis may occur. • Myocardial toxicity with CHF may occur during therapy or following therapy. Cumulative doses greater than 900 mg/m^2 should not be exceeded. • Alopecia is complete with hair regrowth in 2–3 months. • Hyperpigmentation of nail beds and dermal

ETOPOSIDE (VePesid, VP-16)

Dosage:
- 50-100 mg/m² IV qd × 5 (testicular cancer) q 3-4 wk
- 75-200 mg/m² IV qd × 3 (small cell lung cancer) q 3-4 wk. Oral dose is twice the intravenous dose.
- 400 mg/m²/day × 3 days prior to bone marrow transplant.

Efficacy:
- Small cell lung cancer
- Testicular cancer

Mechanism of action:
- Inhibits DNA synthesis in S and G₂. Causes single-strand breaks in DNA.
- Cell-cycle phase specific for S and G₂ phase.

Metabolism:
- Extensively protein bound. Metabolized in the liver. Excreted in the bile and urine
- t½ = 8-14 hr

Administration precautions:
- Following dilution in NS or 5% dextrose, the drug is stable for 72-96 hr at room temperature. At room temperature, stability is dependent on concentration:
  - .6 mg/mL = 24 hr
  - 1 mg/mL = 4 hr
  - 2 mg/mL = 2 hr
- Etoposide is administered slowly over at least 30-45 min.
- Hypotension can occur, monitor patients for drug sensitivity.

creases; dermatitis may occur.
- Radiation recall may occur.
- Red discoloration of urine occurs over 24 hours following drug administration.
- Facial flushing may occur with rapid drug administration.
- Drug is a severe vesicant and should be administered with caution.
- Irreversible amenorrhea may occur in premenopausal women.

Side effects:
- DLT: Leukopenia, dose-related. Nadir occurs 7-14 days, recovery by day 21.
- Nausea and vomiting are uncommon.
- Anorexia occurs, especially with oral dosing.
- Alopecia occurs more commonly with IV dosing. Radiation recall and pruritus can occur.
- HSR reactions are rare.

Appendix 19B Intravenous Antineoplastic Agents (continued)

Dosage and Efficacy	Mechanism of Action and Metabolism	Administration Precautions	Side Effects
	FLUDARABINE (Fludara)		
Dosage: • 25 mg/m² /day × 5 days q 4 week. *Efficacy:* • Chronic lymphocytic leukemia • Low-grade non-Hodgkin's lymphomas	*Mechanism of Action:* • Antimetabolite • Inhibits DNA synthesis *Metabolism:* • Rapidly metabolized to its active form when given intravenously. • t ½ life is 10 hours. • Major route of elimination is the kidneys. • Approximately 20% of the drug is eliminated unchanged in the urine. • A 30% decrease in dose is suggested for patients with renal dysfunction (creatinine >1.5 mg/dL).	*Administration precautions:* • Reconstitute with sterile water for injection USP 2 ml = 25 mg/ml. Further dilute in 100 ml of Dextrose of 0.9% Sodium Chloride. • Administer of 30 minutes. • Once reconstituted, the drug should be used within 8 hours. • Do not administer with pentostatin.	*Side effects:* • Severe and cumulative bone marrow depression may occur; nadir occurs at 13 days. • Nausea and vomiting are uncommon. • Alopecia is mild. • Elevated SGOT may occur. • Somnolence, fatigue, and peripheral neuropathy with delayed CNS toxicities may occur, especially with higher doses.
	5-FLUOROURACIL (5-FU, Adrucil)		
Dosage: • Doses vary: 300-600 mg/m² IV × 5 days q 3-4 wk • 450-600 mg/m² IV weekly	*Mechanism of action:* • Inhibits the formation of thymidine, which is necessary for DNA synthesis. Causes abnormal RNA synthesis. Acts synergistically with	*Administration precautions:* • May be given a variety of ways: IV as a continuous infusion, IV push, arterial infusion, intracavitary, or intraperitoneally.	*Side effects:* • Mylosuppression may be dose-limiting, but less common with continuous infusion. • Mucositis is most common DLT with continu-

- 800-1200 mg/m^2 continuous infusion × 14-21 days to toxicity

Efficacy:

- Cancer of the breast, colon, rectum, pancreas, stomach, head and neck

methotrexate.

- Cell-cycle phase specific for the S-phase.

Metabolism:

- Poorly absorbed by mouth. After IV administration, the drug is metabolized to active metabolites.
- Approximately 45% of the drug is metabolized by the liver.
- 15% is eliminated unchanged in the urine.
- t ½ = 10-20 min

ous infusions. Symptoms of erythema, soreness, and ulceration may begin within 5-8 days of therapy. Sucking on ice chips as tolerated may decrease oral stomatitis. Diarrhea can be severe, even life threatening, especially when 5-FU is given in higher doses with leucovorin.

- Nausea, vomiting, and anorexia occur less frequently, but are more common when 5-FU is given simultaneously with radiation to the abdomen.
- Skin and nail bed changes occur, especially with continuous infusion. Partial nail loss can occur as well as banding. Palmar-plantar erythrodysesthesias can be severe, necessitating dose reduction and treatment delays. Hyperpigmentation and photosensitivity are common. Patients are cautioned to protect themselves from the sun. Excessive lacrimation due to tear duct stenosis and blurred vision occur in about 25% of patients.
- Headache, cerebellar ataxia, nystagmus, and confusion occur with higher doses.
- Administering 5-FU based on the patient's circadian rhythm may lessen toxicity in general.

- Store at room temperature and protect from light.
- Incompatible with daunorubicin, doxorubicin, idarubicin, cisplatin, cytarabine, and diazepam.
- Compatible with vincristine, methotrexate, potassium chloride, and magnesium sulfate.

Appendix 19B Intravenous Antineoplastic Agents (continued)

Dosage and Efficacy	Mechanism of Action and Metabolism	Administration Precautions	Side Effects
			• Alopecia is dose dependent. • Ataxia occurs in elderly patients. Other CNS changes include headache, drowsiness, and blurred vision.

FLOXURIDINE (FUDR, 5-FUDR)

Dosage and Efficacy	Mechanism of Action and Metabolism	Administration Precautions	Side Effects
Dosage: • 0.1–0.6 mg/kg/day by intrahepatic infusion. Therapy is continued to toxicity, usually 7–14 days. • Circadian infusion protocols have been used. • Intravenous doses range from 0.5–1.0 mg/kg/day for up to 2 weeks by continuous infusion. *Efficacy:* • Adenocarcinoma metastatic to the liver	*Mechanism of action:* • Antimetabolite, similar to 5-FU, interrupts DNA synthesis causing cell death. Cell-cycle phase specific for the S-phase. *Metabolism:* • Metabolized to 5-FU when given IV. • 70%–90% of the drug is metabolized by the liver, and metabolites are excreted by the kidneys and lungs. When given, intrahepatic FUDR has a much higher first pass extraction rate compared to 5-FU and therefore the cytotoxic effect is more localized to the liver. • $t\frac{1}{2} = 0.3$–3.6 hr	*Administration precautions:* • Caution should be exercised as both 5-FU and floxuridine (also called 5-FUDR) are supplied in 500-mg vials and the doses of each are dramatically different. With such similar names it is important to note that mistaking 500 mg of FUDR for 500 mg of 5-FU could be lethal. • FUDR 500-mg vial of lyophilized powder is reconstituted with sterile water. • Generally given via an intraarterial infusion pump • Heparin is added to the FUDR to prevent clotting of the catheter due to the slow infusion rate.	*Side effects:* • When given as an intraarterial infusion an H2 antihistamine such as ranitidine may be recommended (150 mg bid) to prevent peptic ulcer disease. • The intraarterial route is usually associated with less systemic toxicity. • Bone marrow suppression is more common with IV bolus injections. • Nausea, vomiting, and anorexia are common. Abdominal cramps with severe diarrhea are indications to interrupt therapy. • Mucositis does not occur often and if it occurs is an indication to interrupt the treatment and to reduce the dose.

GEMCITABINE (Gemzar)

Dosage:
- 800–1000 mg/^{2} weekly × 3 weeks q 4 wk

Efficacy:
- Pancreas cancer
- Non-small cell lung cancer
- Breast cancer

Mechanism of action:
- Antimetabolite
- Inhibits DNA synthesis
- Cell-cycle specific for the S-phase

Metabolism:
- Eliminated by kidneys
- t ½ = 20 min

Administration precautions:
- Reconstitute with sodium chloride to a solution containing 10 mg/mL.
- Dilute in 100–1000 mL of saline and infuse over 30 min to 3 hr.

- Skin changes can occur and include edema, dermatitis, rashes, and pruritus as well as hyperpigmentation.
- Alopecia can occur but is usually mild.

Side effects:
- Myelosuppression, especially thrombocytopenia, can be dose-limiting.
- Flulike syndrome with fever, mild nausea, and vomiting can occur. Fever generally occurs within 8 hr of dosing. Acetaminophen generally relieves symptoms.
- Rash may occur within 2–3 days of the infusion. Topical steroids may be helpful.
- Peripheral edema may occur.

IDARUBICIN (Idamycin)

Dosage:
- 12 mg/m^2/day × 3 days
- Doses vary
- Generally given in combination with other drugs

Mechanism of action:
- Cell-cycle phase specific for S-phase
- Analog of daunorubicin
- Inhibits RNA synthesis

Administration precautions:
- Reconstituted with NS.
- Protect from light.
- Caution is used during administration because drug is a vesicant.

Side effects:
- DLT: Leukopenia and thrombocytopenia are expected.
- Urine can be pink to red for 48 hr after administration.

Appendix 19B Intravenous Antineoplastic Agents (continued)

Dosage and Efficacy	Mechanism of Action and Metabolism	Administration Precautions	Side Effects
Efficacy:	*Metabolism:*	• Incompatible with 5-FU, etoposide, dexamethasone, heparin, hydrocortisone, methotrexate, and vincristine.	• Nausea can be mild to moderate and preventable with standard antiemetic.
• Acute nonlymphocytic leukemia	• Excreted primarily in the bile and urine		• Diarrhea and mucositis can occur.
	• 25% of the drug is eliminated over approximately 5 days		• Alopecia occurs gradually.
	• t ½ = 13–26 hr		• Cumulative cardiomyopathy and CHF can occur with large cumulative doses.
	• Metabolized in the liver to active form		

IFOSFAMIDE (Ifex)

Dosage:	*Mechanism of action:*	*Administration precautions:*	*Side effects:*
• IV: 1.0–1.2 g/m²/day over a 5-day period q 3–4 wk. Higher doses of 2.5–3.7 g/m²/day over a 2- to 3-day period.	• Ifosfamide is an alkylating agent. It is a prodrug and requires activation in the liver by microsomal enzymes.	• Ifosfamide is administered over at least 30 min with aggressive hydration to reduce the incidence of hemorrhagic cystitis.	• Myelosuppression is the DLT.
			• WBC nadir usually occurs 7–10 days posttreatment.
• Mesna at a dose of 20% of the ifosfamide dose is given just prior to the ifosfamide and q 4 h for 2 more doses. Mesna may be given IV or PO.	*Metabolism:*	• The uroprotectant mesna is also given either as a continuous infusion or in divided doses q 4 h × 3 doses.	• Urinary tract toxicity is the dose-limiting toxicity and is manifested as hemorrhagic cystitis. Patients may complain of dysuria and frequency 2–3 days after the infusion. Encourage oral intake of 2–3 L per day prior to and after dosing. Encourage patients to empty their bladders every 2–3 hr.
	• Metabolized by the liver to inactive metabolites.		
	• 15%–56% of the drug is excreted unchanged in the urine.	• Ifosfamide and mesna are compatible and can be infused concurrently when high-dose ifosfamide is given.	
Efficacy:	• t ½ = 7–15 hr		
• Testicular cancer	• Drug elimination may be hindered by renal dysfunction.		• Nausea and vomiting are common with higher doses. Symptoms are preventable with
• Soft tissue sarcoma			
• Hodgkin's and non-Hodgkin's lymphoma			

- Acute leukemias
- Ewing's sarcoma
- Osteosarcoma

- serotonin antagonist therapy.
- Avoid sedation with neurotoxic drugs that can exacerbate the lethargy and confusion that can occur due to the accumulation of chloroacetylaldehyde, a metabolite with neurotoxic properties.
- Alopecia is more common with higher doses and occurs usually within 3 wk of therapy.

IRINOTECAN (Camptosar, CPT-11)

Dosage:
- 125-150 mg/m² IV over 90 min weekly × 4 wk q 6 wk

Efficacy:
- Adenocarcinoma
- Colon/rectal cancer

Mechanism of action:
- Topoisomerase I inhibitor
- Blocks DNA and RNA synthesis in dividing cells

Metabolism:
- Metabolized to its active form in liver
- 20% drug excreted in urine
- 30% excreted in bile
- t½ = 6-10 hr

Administration precautions:
- Dilute in 5% dextrose: stable for 24 hr at room temperature.
- Drug is an irritant.

Side effects:
- Dose-limiting toxicities are diarrhea and myelosuppression.
- Loperamide is administered for diarrhea.
- Flushing and diaphoresis may occur during infusion.
- Moderate to severe nausea and vomiting may occur.

L-ASPARAGINASE (Elspar) Erwinia Asparaginase

Dosage:
- Used in combination with other drugs, active

Mechanism of action:
- Inhibits protein synthesis

Administration precautions:
- Dilute in nonpreserved sterile saline or water.

Side effects:
- Anaphylactic reactions can occur in 20%-35%

PART VII

407

Appendix 19B Intravenous Antineoplastic Agents (continued)

Dosage and Efficacy	Mechanism of Action and Metabolism	Administration Precautions	Side Effects
in ALL 200 IU/day for 28 days, 1000 IU/kg × 10 days or • 20,000 IU/m²/wk *Efficacy:* • ALL	*Metabolism:* • Biphasic elimination • t 1/2 = 4–9 hr and 1.4–1.8 days • Binds to vascular binding sites • May be eliminated by the liver	*Use within 8 hr.* • Refrigerate before and after reconstitution. • Do not infuse through a filter. • IV slow push over 30 min, or IM. • Do not use if solution is cloudy. • Skin test with 2 IU intradermal at least 1 hr prior to dosing. • Administer subsequent doses with caution despite negative skin test.	of patients. • Monitor closely with appropriate support. • IM use is associated with delayed allergic response. • If HSR occurs, the Erwinia preparation may be used with prophylactic premedication. • Urticarial eruptions are common. • Incidence of reactions increases with each subsequent dosing. • Slight anemia can occur; leukopenia is rare. • Malaise, anorexia, nausea, and vomiting occur frequently. • Hepatic toxicity is uncommon. • Lethargy, somnolence, disorientation, and loss of recent memory occur with higher doses.

MECHLORETHAMINE HYDROCHLORIDE (nitrogen mustard, Mustargen)

Dosage and Efficacy	Mechanism of Action and Metabolism	Administration Precautions	Side Effects
Dosage: • IV: 6 mg/m² on days 1 and 8 • Topically: 10 mg/60 mL ointment	*Mechanism of action:* • Alkylating agent results in abnormal base pairing causing DNA miscoding, cross-linking of DNA, and strand breakage.	*Administration precautions:* • Once reconstituted with sterile water or NS the drug should be used within 60 min because of its instability.	*Side effects:* • Myelosuppression is the DLI. • Leukopenia occurs 8–14 days following treatment. Severe thrombocytopenia may occur.

Efficacy:
- Hodgkin's disease
- CML
- Lymphosarcoma

- Cell-cycle nonspecific

Metabolism:
- Rapidly deactivated in the blood
- t½ = 15 min

- Nitrogen mustard should be administered by IV push via a freely running IV line.
- Administering nitrogen mustard via direct IV push technique can cause venous thrombosis and pain.
- Nitrogen mustard is a severe vesicant and must be given with extreme caution.
- Assess for a blood return every 1 mL of injection.
- If extravasation occurs, inject a solution of sodium thiosulfate (1/6 molar) into the area to neutralize the drug.
- For 1 mg of nitrogen mustard infiltrated, inject 2 mL of the 10% thiosulfate solution.
- Preparation: 4 mL sodium thiosulfate injection (10%) diluted with 6 mL of sterile water for injection.

- Severe nausea and vomiting within 1 hr of IV administration. Patients should be premedicated with aggressive antiemetic therapy.
- Alopecia is common. A metallic taste is common during the injection and can be masked by encouraging the patient to chew gum or bite on a lemon rind.
- Amenorrhea and impaired spermatogenesis occurs and is dose dependent.

MELPHALAN (Alkeran, L-PAM, L-Phenylalanine Mustard)

Dosage:
- IV: 16 mg/m² q 3 wk × 4 doses then q 4 wk
- PO: 2 mg/kg/day × 5 days q 4-6 wk
- BMT: 50-60 mg/m² IV

Mechanism of action:
- Alkylating agent; cycle specific
- Forms DNA cross-links

Metabolism:
- 80%-90% of the drug is bound to plasma

Administration precautions:
- Reconstitute with 10 mL of supplied diluent for a concentration = 5 mg/mL.
- Dilute in NS to a concentration of 0.45 mg/mL and use within 60 min.

Side effects:
- Myelosuppression is the DLT.
- GI: mild anorexia, nausea and vomiting when taken orally. Nausea and vomiting can be severe with higher IV doses. Mucositis, diarrhea,

Appendix 19B Intravenous Antineoplastic Agents (continued)

Dosage and Efficacy	Mechanism of Action and Metabolism	Administration Precautions	Side Effects
Efficacy: • Multiple myeloma • Epithelial carcinoma of the ovary • BMT	proteins • 10%–15% of the drug is eliminated unchanged in the urine • t ½ = 1.5–4.0 hr	• Do not refrigerate reconstituted product. • When taken orally, peak plasma levels are reached within 2 hr. The drug is poorly absorbed when taken with food.	and oral ulceration occur infrequently. Leukopenia and thrombocytopenia peak at 2–3 wk and may be cumulative with a prolonged recovery period of 6 or more wk. • Pruritus, dermatitis, and rash may occur. Alopecia is not common with oral dosing. • Amenorrhea and oligospermia are common. • Second malignancies (leukemias) have been reported.
METHOTREXATE (MTX, Mexate, amethopterin)			
Dosage: • 15–30 mg/day × 5 days or 20–30 mg/m² twice weekly • Single doses of 1.5–20 g/m² with leucovorin rescue • Intrathecal dosing 10–15 mg in 7–15 mL of preservative-free saline *Efficacy:* • Trophoblastic neoplasms	*Mechanism of action:* • MTX tightly binds to dihydrofolate reductase thereby blocking the reduction of dihydrofolate to tetrahydrofolic acid, the active form of folic acid. This process effectively arrests DNA, RNA, and protein synthesis. • Antimetabolite • Cell-cycle specific for the S-phase of the cell cycle	*Administration precautions:* • Lower doses (< 100 mg) are usually given IVP without leucovorin rescue. • When given with 5-FU for breast cancer, the MTX dose is followed in 1 hr by the 5-FU. The drugs is synergistic when given this way. • Leucovorin rescue is needed because the dose of MTX is generally > 100 mg. • Preservative-free MTX used for intrathecal injection should be prepared just prior to use.	*Side effects:* • Myelosuppression is the DLT. Leukopenia is dose-dependent and is more likely to occur with prolonged exposure. • Nausea and vomiting are common with higher doses. Diarrhea can be dose limiting. Stomatitis is more common with higher doses and more lengthy infusions. • Skin erythema, hyperpigmentation, photosensitivity, rash, folliculitis, and pruritus may

- Acute leukemias
- Meningeal leukemias
- Carcinoma of the breast
- Osteogenic sarcoma
- Burkitt's lymphoma

Metabolism:

- MTX is distributed freely in water, which means that it will circulate in third space fluid, increasing the toxicity of the drug since it is not being metabolized. Patients with effusions or ascites should be monitored carefully to avoid severe toxicity.
- MTX is highly protein bound and should not be given with acids that may compete for binding (elimination) sites, which would increase the AUC of the MTX, resulting in extreme toxicity.
- 90% of MTX is eliminated from the kidneys in the urine as unchanged drug.
- BUN and creatinine levels should be monitored regularly. If there is evidence of renal impairment lower doses should be given with leucovorin rescue.

- Protect infusions from light.

occur. MTX can cause enhanced radiation side effects if given simultaneously.
- Renal dysfunction is dose-related and more common in patients who are dehydrated. When given in higher doses, the patient's urine pH must be >7 to prevent precipitation of the MTX in the renal tubules, with subsequent renal damage. Administer bicarb as directed. The BUN and creatinine are monitored prior to high-dose therapy.
- Neurological dysfunction can occur with intrathecal administration, especially if cranial radiation has also been given.
- Photophobia, excessive lacrimation, and conjunctivitis have been noted.

MITOMYCIN (Mutamycin, mitomycin C)

Dosage:

- 20 mg/m² as a single dose repeated q 6-8 wk
- For bladder instillation: 20-40 mg is mixed with 20-40 mL of water or saline and is given q 1-2 wk

Mechanism of action:

- Antitumor antibiotic
- Active during the G_1 and S-phase of the cell cycle
- Disrupts DNA synthesis secondary to alkylation

Administration precautions:

- Reconstitute in sterile water: 10 mL in 5 mg vial = 0.5 mg/mL. Use within 3 hr.
- Mitomycin is a severe vesicant. Administer with caution.

Side effects:

- Myelosuppression is the DLT.
- Leukopenia and thrombocytopenia occur late at 4-5 wk with recovery at 7-8 wk. Both are cumulative.

Appendix 19B Intravenous Antineoplastic Agents (continued)

Dosage and Efficacy	Mechanism of Action and Metabolism	Administration Precautions	Side Effects
Efficacy: • Adenocarcinoma of the stomach, pancreas • Cancer of the bladder, breast	*Metabolism:* • Mitomycin is inactivated by microsomal enzymes in the liver and is metabolized in the spleen and kidneys. • 10%–30% of the drug is eliminated unchanged in the urine • $t \frac{1}{2} = 0.5$–1.0 hr	• Give IV push through the side arm of a freely running IV to minimize venous irritation. Assess for a blood return every 1 mL of drug. Discontinue the injection immediately if the patient complains of pain or burning. • Mitomycin can cause tissue damage without evidence of drug infiltration. • Skin ulceration may occur at sites distant from the site of drug administration.	• Anemia and hemolytic-uremic syndrome have been reported. • Nausea and vomiting are mild. • Alopecia is mild, photosensitivity, skin rash, and pruritus are uncommon. • Venoocclusive disease of the liver with abdominal pain, hepatomegaly, and liver failure occur in patients receiving mitomycin and BMT. • Pulmonary fibrosis has been reported.
MITOXANTRONE (Novantrone)			
Dosage: • 10–12 mg/m²/day × 5 days for induction of acute nonlymphocytic leukemia; 12 mg/m² q 3–4 wk *Efficacy:* • Acute monocytic leukemia • AML • Acute promyelocytic leukemia	*Mechanism of action:* • Antitumor antibiotic • Intercalates into DNA; disrupts cell division *Metabolism:* • Metabolized in the liver and excreted in the bile and urine • $t \frac{1}{2} = 24$–37 hr	*Administration precautions:* • Dark blue solution in vials • Dilute in at least 50 mL D5W or NS. • Stable for 7 days at room temperature. • Administer IV over at least 5 min as an infusion.	*Side effects:* • Leukopenia is the DLT. • Nausea and vomiting are mild and preventable. Alopecia is common. Diarrhea and stomatitis may occur. • Cumulative cardiomyopathy can occur. Monitoring the left ventricular ejection fraction is indicated, especially in patients who are at risk for heart disease or who have received

- Breast cancer
- Primary hepatocellular carcinoma

doxorubicin in the past.
- Blue discoloration of the sclera may occur. The urine may remain blue-green for 48 hr following treatment.

PACLITAXEL (Taxol)

Dosage:	*Mechanism of action:*	*Administration precautions:*	*Side effects:*
• 200-250 mg/m² q 3 wk or in heavily pre-treated patients	• Promotes assembly of microtubules and stabilizes them, thereby blocking mitosis.	• Formulated in 50% polyoxyethylated castor oil ((Cremophor EL) and 50% dehydrated alcohol.	• HSRs occur infrequently with proper premedication. Most HSRs occur within the first or second dosing. Symptoms include dyspnea, urticaria, flushing, and hypotension.
• 135-170 mg/m² q 3 wk or weekly in divided doses	• Paclitaxel also prevents transition of the cell from G₀ phase to S phase by blocking cellular response to growth factors.	• Administer only in glass bottles or non-PVC containers (polyolefin containers using polyethylene-lined nitroglycerin tubing sets).	• DLI is myelosuppression.
Efficacy:	*Metabolism:*	• Cremophor-containing solutions will leach the plasticizer DEHP from PVC containers.	• Leukopenic nadir occurs 7-10 days after dosing, with recovery at 15 days. Anemia and thrombocytopenia occur less frequently.
• Ovarian carcinoma	• The majority of paclitaxel is protein bound.	DEHP can cause liver toxicity.	• Peripheral neuropathy occurs more commonly in patients who are also receiving cisplatin. Hyperesthesias and burning pain in the feet may also occur. Myalgias and arthralgias occur usually 3-4 days after dosing.
• Breast cancer	• Elimination is primarily hepatic; minimal renal excretion	• Inline filtration is needed (.02 μm) due to the natural origins of the drug.	
• Non-small cell lung cancer	• t½ = 1.3-8.0 hr	• Administration rate varies from 1-3 hr to 24-96 hr. In general, the longer the infusion, the more likely the patient will experience myelosuppression that is dose limiting.	• Vioxx or Celebrex may be effective to minimize myalgias.
		• Hypersensitivity reactions can occur with paclitaxel infusion and are thought to be re-	• Alopecia is complete at 3 wk.
			• Mucositis occurs more commonly with pro-

Dosage and Efficacy	Mechanism of Action and Metabolism	Administration Precautions	Side Effects
		lated to the Cremophor EL. Patients are premedicated with dexamethasone 20 mg at 13 and 7 hr prior to treatment; with diphenhydramine 50 mg IV 30 min prior, and with an H_2 blocker (cimetidine 300 mg or pepcid 20 mg) 30 min prior. • When administering paclitaxel with doxorubicin, the doxorubicin is given first; likewise when paclitaxel is given with cisplatin or carboplatin, the paclitaxel is given first to avoid disruption in the elimination of the platinum compound and enhanced toxicity. • Synergistic with herceptin.	longed infusions. Nausea and vomiting are mild. Diarrhea occurs infrequently. Paclitaxel is an irritant but can cause blistering and skin breakdown if large amounts of more concentrated drug are infiltrated.

RITUXIMAB (Rituxan)

Dosage and Efficacy	Mechanism of Action and Metabolism	Administration Precautions	Side Effects
Dosage: • 375mg/m² given as IV infusion weekly for 4 weeks *Efficacy:* • Relapsed or refractory low-grade or follicular,	*Mechanism of action:* • A monoclonal antibody that is genetically engineered and directed against the CD 20 antigen found on the surface of B-cell lymphocytes	*Administration precautions:* • Protect vials from direct sunlight. • Dose is added to 0.9% Sodium Chloride USP or 5% Dextrose, resulting in a final concentration of 1–4 mg/mL.	*Side effects:* • Hypersensitivity reactions are common; hypotension, brochospasm, and angioedema may occur. • Treat with diphenhydramine and acetamino-

CD20 positive, B-cell non-Hodgkin's lymphoma

- The rituximab CD20 binds to the CD 20 antigen on B lymphocytes with lysis of the B lymphocyte.

Metabolism:
- Median serum half life ranges from 60–174 hours.
- Drug may be detected in serum up to 3–6 months after treatment.

- Drug is stable in infusion for 24 hours at 2–8 degrees C and at room temperature for 36 hours.
- Initial infusion rate is 50 mg/hr; if no hypersensitivity or infusion-related problems, increase the infusion rate 50 mg/hr every 30 minutes to a maximum of 400 mg/hr.
- If reaction occurs, slow or stop the infusion. May continue the infusion at one half of the previous rate.
- Subsequent infusions: infuse at 100 mg/hr; increase by 100 mg/hr every 30 minutes.
- Do not administer as an intravenous push.
- Cardiac monitoring during and after infusions are indicated if cardiac arrythmias occur.

phen; bronchodilators, epinephrine, or IV saline are used.
- Infusion-related reactions occur within 30 minutes to 2 hours of the infusion. Fever and chills/rigors affect most patients during the first infusion.
- Nausea, urticaria, fatigue, headache, pruritus, bronchospasm, dyspnea, hypotension, flushing, and pain at the disease site have been reported.
- Severe myelosuppresion has been reported.
- tumor lysis syndrome can occur in patients with a heavy tumor load. Monitor serum electrolytes and renal function.

TENIPOSIDE (Vumon, VM-26)

Dosage:
- 100 mg/m² 1-2 times weekly and 20-60 mg/m² × 5 days or 90 mg/m²/day × 5 days for lung cancer

Efficacy:
- Relapsed or refractory acute lymphoblastic

Mechanism of action:
- Plant alkaloid, topoisomerase II inhibitor
- Phase specific, acts in late S phase and early G₂ phase

Metabolism:
- Bound to plasma protein; metabolized in the

Administration precautions:
- Dosage is diluted in sodium chloride and is physically stable for approximately 24 hr at room temperature in glass containers. Drug may precipitate in plastic containers.
- Administer over at least a 45-min period to avoid severe hypotension.

Side effects:
- Leukopenia is the DLT occurring at 10-14 days.
- Nausea and vomiting are rare.
- Alopecia occurs gradually; skin rash is rare.
- With high-dose therapy, severe skin rashes can occur.

Appendix 19B Intravenous Antineoplastic Agents (continued)

Dosage and Efficacy	Mechanism of Action and Metabolism	Administration Precautions	Side Effects
leukemia • Small cell lung cancer	liver with less than 10% of the unchanged drug in feces • Eliminated in the urine • t ½ = 20 hr	• Avoid extravasation. • Local phlebitis may occur. • HSRs occur and include blood pressure changes, bronchospasm, tachycardia, urticaria, facial flushing, diaphoresis, periorbital edema, vomiting, and/or fever.	• Hemolytic anemia with renal failure has occurred. • HSR may be related to the Cremophor EL vehicle. • Secondary malignancies occur infrequently. • Hyperbilirubinemia, SGOT, and SGPT elevations can occur.
THIOTEPA (Thioplex)			
Dosage: • 12–16 mg/m² q 1–4 wk • 900 mg/m² (transplant dose) • 30–60 mg q wk × 4 wk for intravesicular use • 1.0–10 mg/m² 1–2 times per wk for intrathecal use *Efficacy:* • Breast cancer • Ovarian cancer • Superficial bladder cancer • Lymphoma • Hodgkin's disease	*Mechanism of action:* • An alkylating agent similiar to nitrogen mustard *Metabolism:* • Variably absorbed through the bladder mucosa following intravesical injection • Metabolized in the liver • t ½ = 2–3 hr	*Administration precautions:* • 15-mg vial is reconstituted with 1.5 mL of sterile water and further diluted with saline for intrathecal use (preservative free). • Intravenous and intravesical solutions may be diluted with saline, D5W, or lactated Ringer's solution and are chemically stable for at least 5 days in the refrigerator and 24 hr at room temperature. • Intravesical instillation involves placement of a catheter in the bladder and instillation of the drug with retention of the liquid for up to	*Side effects:* • Myelosuppression is the DLI and may be cumulative. • Leukopenia occurs 7–10 days postinjection. • Thrombocytopenia may be delayed. • Nausea and vomiting are not common in nontransplant doses. • Stomatitis may be severe in transplant doses. • Abdominal pain, hematuria, dysuria, frequency, and urgency occur with intravesical instillation. • Second malignancies have been reported.

2 hr. The patient is repositioned q 15 min to maximize exposure to the tissues of the bladder.

- Intrathecal doses are mixed in up to 20 mL of Ringer's lactate to maximize CNS distribution.
- Intravenous administration may be given IVP or as an infusion. Thiotepa is not a vesicant.

TOPOTECAN (Hycamtin)

Dosage:	*Mechanism of action:*	*Administration precautions:*	*Side effects:*
• 1.3–1.6 mg/m^2 IV infusion over 30 min, 2 hr, or 24 hr or • 1.5–2.0 mg/m^2/day as a 30-min infusion × 5 days *Efficacy:* • Small cell lung cancer • Ovarian cancer • Esophageal cancer	• Topoisomerase I inhibitor causes single strand breaks in DNA, causing the cell to die during DNA replication *Metabolism:* • Up to 48% of the drug is eliminated unchanged in the urine • t½ = 3 hr	• 5-mg vial is reconstituted with 2 mL of sterile water and diluted in D5W. • Stable for up to 48 hr at room temperature. • Given intravenously as an infusion.	• Leukopenia is the DLI, and the nadir occurs at day 10–12 with recovery at 3 wk. • Thrombocytopenia and anemia occur but are not usually dose limiting. • Mild to moderate nausea and vomiting may occur. Diarrhea has been reported to occur during or shortly after the infusion. • Fever and mild flulike symptoms are reported. • Alopecia and skin rash may occur. • Elevated LFTs are common. • Headache, dizziness, lightheadedness, and peripheral neuropathy have been reported.

Dosage and Efficacy	Mechanism of Action and Metabolism	Administration Precautions	Side Effects
	TRASGUZUMAB (Herceptin)		
Dosage: • Loading dose: 4 mg/kg IV week 1 • Maintenance dose: 2 mg/kg IV weekly beginning week 2 • Alternative dosing schedule: 6 mg/kg IV every three weeks *Efficacy:* • Breast cancer: 25% of women with breast cancer over-express the human epidermal growth factor receptor.	*Mechanism of action:* • Hereptin is thought to antagonize the function of the growth-signaling properties of the HER-2 gene. It signals immune cells to attack and kiss malignant cells that overexpress the HER-2 protein. *Metabolism:* • Mean half life is upo three weeks • Metabolized in the liver	*Administration precautions:* • Reconstitute with 20 ml of Bacteriostatic water for injection. Do Not Shake. further dilute desired dose (22 mg/ml) in 250 ml of 0.9% Sodium Chloride injection. • Drug is stable for 28 days following reconstitution at 2–8 degrees C. • First administration is given over 90 minutes with a 60-minute observation period. • Subsequent infusions are given over 30 minutes. • Monitor vitals every 15 minutes during the first infusion. • Observe for allergic reactions: Administer diphenhydramine and acetaminophen in the event of an allergic reaction. • Fever, chills, and body aches are common. Slow the infusion, monitor the patient, and reinstitute the infusion following resolution of the above symptoms.	*Side effects:* • Ventricular dysfunction and congestive heart failure are major complications, especially if the patient has received doxorubicin in the past or has a history of hear failure. • Patients are evaluated frequently with muga scans and baseline cardiac function.

418

VINBLASTINE (Velban)

Dosage:

- 6-10 mg/m² q 2-4 wk; 1.7-2.0 mg/m²/day weekly as a continuous infusion or over a period of 96 hr

Efficacy:

- Hodgkin's disease
- Non-Hodgkin's lymphoma
- Testicular cancer
- Kaposi's sarcoma
- Breast cancer
- Melanoma
- Cancers of the kidney, bladder, and cervix
- Head and neck cancers
- Lung cancer
- Ovarian cancer

Mechanism of action:

- Cell-cycle phase specific for the M phase
- A plant alkaloid that binds to tubulin causing inhibition of the microtubule assembly, which inhibits mitotic spindle formation.

Metabolism:

- Metabolized by the liver
- Less than 1% is eliminated unchanged in the urine
- t½ = 20 hr

Administration precautions:

- Reconstituted with 10 mL of bacteriostatic NS to yield a concentration of 1 mg/mL.
- Dose may be further diluted with D5W or NS for continuous infusion.
- Continuous infusions may only be given through central lines because vinblastine is a severe vesicant if infiltrated.
- Store in the refrigerator. Stable for 14 days at room temperature and for 30 days under refrigeration.

Side effects:

- Leukopenia is the DLI.
- Thrombocytopenia and anemia are less common.
- Nausea and vomiting, anorexia, diarrhea, and mucositis are rare.
- Peripheral neuropathy, constipation, paralytic ileus, and urinary retention may occur.
- Alopecia occurs with higher doses.
- Rash and photosensitivity may occur.
- Infiltration may cause ulceration depending on the amount of drug extravasated.
- Treatment with hyaluronidase and heat may minimize ulceration.
- Incompatible with heparin and furosemide.
- Compatible in solution with doxorubicin, metoclopramide, dacarbazine, and bleomycin.

Appendix 19B Intravenous Antineoplastic Agents (continued)

Dosage and Efficacy	Mechanism of Action and Metabolism	Administration Precautions	Side Effects
	VINCRISTINE (Oncovin)		
Dosage:	*Mechanism of action:*	*Administration precautions:*	*Side effects:*
• 0.5–1.4 mg/m² q 1–4 wk	• Plant alkaloid	• Store in the refrigerator.	• Myelosuppression is mild. Nausea, vomiting, anorexia, and diarrhea are rare.
• Continuous infusion regimens of 0.5 mg/day to 0.5 mg/m²/day × 4 days may be used.	• Binds to tubulin, causing inhibition of microtubule assembly, which inhibits mitotic spindle formation	• Stable for at least 30 days at room temperature.	
		• Doses for continuous infusion are further diluted with NS or D5W.	• Constipation and abdominal pain may occur due to the neurological toxicity of the drug.
Efficacy:	• M phase specific.	• Compatible with doxorubicin, bleomycin, cytarabine, fluorouracil, methotrexate, and metoclopramide.	• Prophylactic stool softeners and laxatives may be indicated in patients at high risk for constipation.
• Acute leukemia	*Metabolism:*		
• Hodgkin's disease	• Metabolized by the liver.	• Vincristine is a vesicant that should be given with caution and through a central line when given as a continuous infusion.	• Alopecia is minimal. Paresthesias, ataxia, hoarseness, myalgias, headache, and seizures may occur.
• Non–Hodgkin's lymphoma	• 40%–70% excreted in the bile.		
• Rhabdomyosarcoma	• t½ = 70–100 hr	• If infiltration occurs, a ply ice pack for 20 minutes out of every hour for 24 hours.	• Severe pain in the jaw may occur.
• Neuroblastoma		• Greater than 2 mg total dose is usually contraindicated due to the toxicity of the drug.	
• Wilms' tumor		• Vincristine is lethal if given intrathecally and should be labeled as such when dispensed by the pharmacist.	
• Ewing's sarcoma			
• Melanoma		• Administer with caution in patients with obvious liver dysfunction.	
• Multiple myeloma			
• Breast cancer			
• Lung cancer			

420

VINORELBINE TARTRATE (Navelbine)

Dosage:
- PO: 40-mg capsule for oral use
- IV: 30–40 mg/m^2 weekly

Efficacy:
- Breast cancer
- Ovarian cancer
- Head and neck cancer
- Esophageal cancer
- Non-small cell lung cancer
- Lung cancer
- Germ cell cancers
- Hodgkin's disease

Mechanism of action:
- Cell-cycle specific
- Produces cell blockade in G$_2$ and M phase
- Blocks polymerization of microtubules
- Impairs mitotic spindle

Metabolism:
- Hepatic elimination
- Binds to plasma proteins
- Nonrenal elimination

Administration precautions:
- Venous irritation occurs in about 25% of patients. Symptoms include erythema and pain at the site, vein discoloration and tenderness along the vein.
- Administer drug over 6–10 min through the side arm of a freely running IV. Inject through the port farthest from the IV site.
- Follow injection with 75–125 mL of IV fluid to flush the line (peripheral IV sites only).
- Local tissue damage/necrosis, phlebitis may occur if the drug infiltrates.
- Dose reduction may be appropriate for patients with impaired liver function: If bilirubin is >2.1, the dose of vinorelbine is reduced 50%–75% (i.e, 15–7.5 mg/m^2).
- Pain at the tumor site can occur during administration.
- Vinorelbine is compatible with metoclopramide, ondansetron, chlorpromazine, promethazine, and dexamethasone.

Side effects:
- DLT: Noncumulative neutropenia
- Alopecia/hair thinning after several treatments
- Anorexia
- Asthenia
- Peripheral neuropathy
- Constipation occurs in about 1/3 of patients and increases after several treatments.
- Fatigue can be cumulative.
- Arthralgias and myalgias
- Rash (rare)
- Typhlitis with abdominal pain and fever occur 3–4 days after treatment in heavily pretreated patients.
- Jaw pain is rare.

- Vinorelbine is incompatible with 5-FU, thiotepa, furosemide, amphotericin, ampicillin, piperacillin, aminophylline, and sodium bicarbonate.

ALL = acute lymphocytic leukemia; AML = acute myelogenous leukemia; AUC = area under the curve; BMT = bone marrow transplant; CHF = congestive heart failure; CI = continuous infusion; D5W = 5% dextrose in water; DLT = dose-limiting toxicity; 5-FU = fluorouracil; SHT3 = serotonin receptor; GI = gastrointestinal; HSR = hypersensitivity reaction; IM = intramuscular; IP = intraperitoneal; IT = intrathecal; IV = intravenous; IVP = intravenous push; IU = International unit; LFT = liver function test; MUGA = ejection fraction; NS = normal saline; PVC = polyvinyl chloride; QS = quantity sufficient; SIADH = syndrome of inappropriate antidiuretic hormone; SGOT = serum glutamic oxaloacetic transaminase; SGPT = serum glutamic pyruvic transaminase; SQ = subcutaneous; t 1/2 = half-life.

Index